EAT LIKE JESUS

EAT LIKE JESUS

Returning to Kosher Christianity

ANDREW L. HOY

THECLEANEATGREEN.COM

WESTBOW
PRESS
A DIVISION OF THOMAS NELSON

WestBow Press books may be ordered through booksellers or by contacting:

WestBow Press
A Division of Thomas Nelson
1663 Liberty Drive
Bloomington, IN 47403
www.westbowpress.com
1-(866) 928-1240

All Scripture quotations, unless otherwise indicated, are taken from the Holy Bible, New International Version®. NIV®. Copyright © 1973, 1978, 1984 by International Bible Society. Used by permission of Zondervan. All rights reserved.

Footnotes translated from original Aramaic Peshitta texts instead of Greek.

ISBN: 978-1-4497-9129-2 (sc)
ISBN: 978-1-4497-9130-8 (hc)

Library of Congress Control Number: 2013906385

Printed in the United States of America.

WestBow Press rev. date: 05/15/2014

Her priests do violence to my law and profane my holy things; they do not distinguish between the holy and the common; they teach that there is no difference between the unclean and the clean.

—Ezek. 22:26

How can you say, "We are wise, for we have the law of the Lord" when actually the lying pen of the scribes has handled it falsely?

—Jer. 8:8

ACKNOWLEDGEMENTS

The prophet Elihu said, "For I am full of words, and the spirit within me compels me; inside I am like bottled-up wine, like new wineskins ready to burst. I must speak and find relief; I must open my lips and reply. I will show partiality to no one, nor will I flatter any man; for if I were skilled in flattery, my Maker would soon take me away" (Job 32:18-22).

Writing a book is probably among the greatest tests of patience I have ever known. It is a journey defined by ongoing learning and discovery, reflection and introspection, and reconsideration and revision. Like an extended pregnancy, writing can be a prolonged vocation without daily relief. It is to live with full sensory perception and intellect intact—while being denied the ability to be heard. Therefore, I thank my heavenly Father for putting such a spirit of compulsion within me, along with this opportunity to truly "speak" and find relief.

I would also like to express my gratitude to my father and mother for their steadfast support, and to Angie and Julie for their ongoing encouragement. I also thank Johan for colorful comments, Sarah for her voice of reason, Jordan for original inspiration, Henneke for articulate advice, Mark for insightful dialogue, Baruch for kind words of wisdom, Brian for tireless patience, Joe for passion, Jacob for candor, Kay for prompt participation, Sylvie for thoughtful inquiry, and Avram for a spirit of reconciliation, Aubrey for her enthusiasm, and Nathan for his sobering remarks. I thank Ken and Mac for engaging despite their disagreement, and for every pastor along the way willing to entertain my opposition. Finally, I must acknowledge Barb for her insight, and Eric, Marty, Mike, and John for their thoughtful remarks. I beg forgiveness of any friends, family members, and random strangers who have been willing to consider my positions and endure my arguments over the course of the years, whose names I have failed to mention.

TABLE OF CONTENTS

FOREWORD

Although most modern writers use electronic keyboards instead of the reed pens and scribing chisels of Bible times, the prophet Jeremiah's words about the corruption of divine writ remain every bit as relevant today as when they were first proclaimed. Over the course of more than 2,500 years, the only thing that has really changed is the rate at which we can create and multiply errors. Today, working with luxuries such as *backspace* and *delete* keys, inexpensive paper, and virtually unlimited hard drive space, it seems we take these blessings as liberties to think less before typing. As such, our discipline to make each paragraph, each word, and each letter flawless is compromised, for our modern writing tools have removed the incentive to be perfect, contrary to what ancient writing mediums demanded. Hence the need for the second edition of *Eat Like Jesus*.

Given the opening Jeremiah 8:8 citation, it is with a mixture of regret, embarrassment, and irony that I am publishing this second edition, after a reader pointed out what I now believe to be a chronology discrepancy in the second chapter of my first edition. Simply put, I previously assumed a chronology of Peter's vision based on Galatians 2 inferences while overlooking Paul's whereabouts as implied by Acts 9:30 and 11:25 (Paul went to Tarsus to avoid a plot against him). Consequently, Peter's vision was probably not prompted by events in

Antioch, but rather Paul's later rebuke of Peter in Antioch (Galatians 2:11) was necessary because Peter had forgotten the core message conveyed in his own vision—namely that he was to stop alienating God-fearing Gentiles.

Nevertheless, the presumptuous chronology does nothing to undermine the book's overall thesis and conclusions. In fact, my initial assumptions even validate one of the central ideas conveyed throughout EAT LIKE JESUS—that the more we handle Bible texts with preconceived biases, the more likely we are to corrupt the original message. This occasion brings to mind a short poetic proverb, which I faintly recall reading in a scientific publication years ago.

By the questions we pose
ourselves we deceive;
so limited in thought,
by what we choose to perceive.

While a small fraction of my first edition was unduly influenced by my chosen perceptions, I am grateful that the self-deception that resulted was not actually in disagreement with the law of God, to which the sharp opening Jeremiah quotation alludes. Also, I consider myself fortunate in that my questionable assumptions were consistent with Peter's known character shortcomings. The message I glean from Peter's life story is that after making—and even repeating—mistakes, there might remain space for grace, the opportunity for repentance and redemption, and perhaps even the possibility of seeing miracles.

Apart from chapter 2 updates, this edition also incorporates upgrades to chapter 4. Tables were added to enhance presentation of critical Genesis translations, and the corresponding chapter 4 text was revised to better accommodate the new tables.

- Andrew Hoy
Author, Eat Like Jesus
January 2014

ko·sher (adjective)
\\'kō-shər\\

1 a: sanctioned by Jewish law; especially: ritually fit for use
<kosher meat>
b: selling or serving food ritually fit according to Jewish law
<a kosher restaurant>
2: being proper, acceptable, or satisfactory <is the deal
kosher?>

http://www.merriam-webster.com/dictionary/kosher

Chris·tian·i·ty (noun)
\\'kris-chē-'a-nə-tē\\

1: the religion derived from Jesus Christ, based on the
Bible as sacred scripture, and professed by Eastern, Roman
Catholic, and Protestant bodies
2: conformity to the Christian religion

http://www.merriam-webster.com/dictionary/christianity

Perfect in Deed and Perfect in Feed

Christians of all denominations have shared a common belief for centuries. For nearly two thousand years, they have placed their faith—and their eternal destiny—in Jesus' redemptive work. Rather than depending on their own imperfect effort for their eternal salvation, they rely on Jesus' perfect life. Because of this, Christians will zealously attest to Jesus' flawless compliance with all of Moses' law, accepting it as a prerequisite for their salvation.

Given Moses' mandates, it follows that Jesus' righteous status was indeed contingent on what he ate; in other words, Jesus would not have lived a perfect life if he ate things that Moses forbade. The Christian redemption mechanism collapses if Jesus did not keep all of Moses' law, for Christian theology insists that an imperfect sacrifice would fail to meet the Father's expectations. Therefore, Jesus was bound by the entire law or 'Torah' of Moses—including the 'kosher' food laws of Leviticus; Jesus couldn't eat roadkill, blood, or animals slaughtered by strangulation, nor could he eat things like shrimp, lobster, scallops, or swine. Had Jesus eaten such 'foods,' he would have violated Moses' law, disqualifying himself and incurring guilt and sin. Jesus' failure to comply with Moses' food laws would disintegrate the basis for Christian claims of messianic perfection; it would negate his pedigree and render his crucifixion meaningless. For Jesus to be perfect in deed, he had to be perfect in feed.

Eating like Jesus Did—WWJD?

As a matter of obligation, anyone participating in the popular W.W.J.D. (What Would Jesus Do?) movement should investigate the candid gospel testimonies pertaining to all possible facets of Jesus' life—including his diet. The W.W.J.D. question demands that believers research gospel records of Jesus' life to understand what he actually did, lest the acronym embossed on so many bracelets, coffee mugs, and t-shirts amount to nothing more than vain rhetoric. Surveying the gospel texts for food and eating references, people will find that the accounts do not limit Jesus' diet to mere fruits, figs, and grains. In fact, the texts suggest that Jesus ate both fish and lamb; he prepared fish for his disciples[1] and the masses,[2] and he ate the traditional Passover meal with his disciples.[3] On the other hand, gospel writers never describe Jesus as eating unclean foods or animal types forbidden by Moses; there is no evidence that Jesus ever put pork on his fork.

Regardless of the positive sentiments fueling the W.W.J.D. movement, it is not practical or reasonable for people to believe that they can or should emulate Jesus in every way. Gospel texts were obviously not written as fully detailed biographies; thus, it is impossible to know everything that Jesus did. Moreover, many circumstances of modern life do not correlate with those of Jesus' life according to the ancient biblical accounts, making it all the more difficult to do what he did, much less to predict what Jesus would do. Finally, there is the matter of individual identity and purpose; in professing to be the Son of God, Jesus didn't encourage billions of followers to make the same messianic claims as he did. Obviously, God does not expect everyone to turn water into wine, to ride into Jerusalem by donkey, or to curse nearby fig trees.

Eating like Jesus Did—WDJS?

Fortunately, to the benefit of billions of believers, Jesus never instructed his disciples to do exactly as he *did* in gospel texts; instead, he hoped his followers would do exactly as he *said*. Thus a W.D.J.S. (What Did Jesus Say) campaign might be more prudent, since recalling Jesus' imperative instructions is far more practical than speculating W.W.J.D. from incidental gospel accounts. Jesus never said, "Do everything that

1 John 21:9–13
2 Matthew 14:13–21, 15:29–39; Mark 6:30–44, 8:1–13; Luke 9:10–17; John 6:1–15
3 Matthew 26:17–21; Mark 14:12–18; Luke 22:7–16; Exodus 12:3; Numbers 9:11

I do and exactly as I do." Instead he commissioned his followers to *obey* everything that he commanded them.[4] Granted, it may be perfectly reasonable to deduce that Jesus ate only kosher foods based on his messianic obligation to Moses' law and on the ancient gospel descriptions. But it is by far more important for Christians to recall what Jesus *said* about eating and food. After all, clear instructions and imperative statements are generally more effective in communicating divine expectations for humanity than relatively vague examples offered without specific and authoritative language.

But even after carefully examining Jesus' life as described in the four gospel texts, it becomes evident that he said very little about food—and even less about eating. In fact, Jesus never listed types of foods that were acceptable to eat;[5] neither did he list foods that were forbidden to eat. However, it is clear that Jesus had extraordinary reverence for the law of Moses. Jesus repeatedly underscored the divine authority behind Moses' words, and he also touted the eternal validity of Moses' writings.[6] Such statements should logically leave the gospel audience to conclude that Jesus would defer to Moses' law in all dining and dietary affairs. A proper Christian response to a gospel diet study, therefore, might be to inquire, "W.D.M.S.?" (What Did Moses Say?); after all, Jesus made direct reference to Moses' writings on dozens of occasions.

New Testament Food and Dispensational Folly

Nevertheless, a host of popular yet counterfeit Christian doctrines portray Jesus' teachings[7] and New Testament 'food theology' in a radically different light; many Christian institutions even insist that Jesus overturned the dietary laws given through Moses. Such doctrines and teachings can be grouped under the large umbrella of dispensational theology.

---

4 Matthew 28:20
5 Matthew 15:11–20 and Mark 7:15–20 are erroneously inferred as exceptions.
6 e.g., Matthew 5:17–18, 15:3–6; Mark 7:10–13
7 Matthew 15:11, 18–20; Mark 7:15, 18–20

According to dispensational theology, God's commandments and moral expectations for mankind shifted between Old Testament and New Testament eras, or historical "dispensations." Such theology presupposes that New Testament teachings are drastically different in substance and spirit when compared with Old Testament texts, and newer revelations are assumed to replace earlier divine mandates.

While some may perceive a dispensational approach to Bible interpretation to be practical and beneficial on many levels, dispensational theology is wrought with logical complications and carries dangerous implications. First of all, dispensational theologians inherently portray a fickle god—one devoid of stability, without moral absolutes, and with a cheap and pliable notion of justice. Unstable and unpredictable, the dispensationalists' god is perceived as a capricious prankster, making men of certain eras pursue pointless things—including unproductive superstitious rituals—as a result of fear. Since he lacks foreknowledge, the dispensationalists' god is not a competent one and has insufficient control over human history. Instead, this is a god whose rogue creation took him by surprise and thwarted his original plan. This is a god who makes moral standards too unreasonable and too hard to follow, then changes these standards in response to humanity's inability to observe them. Devoid of reason, the dispensationalists' god is a far cry from the one true God, who says, "I change not!"

Dispensational Portraits

Subtly sown dispensational seeds have been scattered throughout all of Christendom and Western society. They sprout in all forms of media, from Sunday sermon series to artistic caricatures in Sunday morning newspaper comics. Where dispensational thinking has taken root, God might be portrayed in Old Testament contexts as an angry old man on a throne, dispatching awful things like plague, famine, and lightning bolts to unequivocally express his wrath. He inspires more fear than love, and he is depicted as an authoritarian deity, pronouncing condemnation over lawbreakers with a stern and intimidating voice.

Unlike the Father or God of the Old Testament, the New Testament Jesus is predominantly portrayed as a benevolent deity within dispensational venues. Jesus is often made out to be a pacifist or peacenik, smiling and lighthearted, mystical and illuminated, full of grace and mercy, often hugging small children and holding little lambs. Unlike an aging and overbearing father, this Jesus can be cool, friendly, and fun. He is depicted as a hero who kept the law for the sake of humanity—so humanity could attain salvation without having to carry such a cumbersome burden or preoccupy itself with such complicated legal detail.

While dispensational doctrine and imagery might vary in its degree or extremity, the effects of dispensational thinking are clearly far-reaching and of great influence. In particular, kosher food laws are treated with indifference and contempt by dispensational theologians—even though such laws were given to humanity for the benefit of human health.

Regardless, dispensational theologians have created an entire 'dining theology' by extrapolating beyond Jesus' teachings and other New Testament accounts, permitting and sometimes even encouraging their congregants to eat defiled or unclean food.[8] This is particularly ironic given the striking parallels between dispensationalism and the New Testament prodigal son[9] parable. After all, it was the rebellious prodigal son who abandoned his father's rules and wound up tending unclean swine in foreign lands!

Christianity Redefined

Nevertheless, as many mainstream Christian institutions have been commandeered by prodigal thinkers, Christianity has been defined according to dispensational standards. In fact, dispensational theology

8 Texts mistranslated and cited out of context to negate Old Testament food laws include Matthew 15:11, 18–20; Mark 7:15, 18–20; Acts 10:15, 11:9; Romans 14:2,14; 1 Corinthians 10:27–31; Colossians 2:20–22.
9 Luke 15:11–32

is the norm in Christian education; it is promoted in Sunday schools, private grade schools, and seminaries, as well as in weekly sermons. Likewise, most religious materials are influenced by dispensational thinking; books, church constitutions, worship liturgy and song, and even Holy Bible translations[10] are replete with dispensational ideas. Consequently, entire Christian congregations are forged into dispensational molds.

But the problem of dispensational precedents predates modern religious institutions and Bible translations; it was not conceived over the course of the latest generation. To the contrary, the public has been saturated with dispensational theology for centuries; and as a result, it is fair to say that Christianity today is no longer a religion defined by its point of origin. Rather than being defined by specific teachings of Jesus or particular Scriptures, Christianity has instead become a religion of creed, human doctrines, and manmade church constitutions. In some cases, it has even become a religion of public opinion.

While it may sound radical to suggest that Christianity has been redefined by public opinion, modern dictionary descriptions testify to the ongoing redefinition of Christianity. According to the dictionary excerpt on the first page of this preface, it is clear that Christianity is somehow defined by secondhand or third-party processing. According to the definition, the words of Christ and sacred writ are not what define the religion; instead, the tenets of Christianity are a matter of *institutional derivation* and *profession*—derivation being a matter of somebody's preference, and profession being a zealous expression of such preference.

But Christianity need not—and must not—be defined or redefined according to the preferences of theologians or in keeping with dispensationalists' worldviews. If Christianity is not defined and constrained exclusively by biblical texts, there is no assurance that the Christianity derived or professed by anyone will be authentic; and

10 The New International Version (NIV) is cited almost exclusively herein, in order to demonstrate dispensational translation biases and the doctrinal implications within Christendom.

if it is not authentic, it must be rejected as something misclassified, mislabeled, or misrepresented. After all, Christianity in a secondhand and institutional sense has been associated with a host of problems, including holy wars, crusades, dictatorial manipulation, political perversions, human traditions, and even choirboy molestation; whereas Christianity in an authentic or fundamental biblical sense cannot be identified as the root cause of such problems.

Defining Kosher Christianity

Because Christianity has been radically redefined by so many different entities, *kosher* and *Christianity* are words unlikely to be found together in religious contexts. Therefore, the term *Kosher Christianity* is likely to be perceived as an oxymoron by Christians and Jews, or possibly even heretical by those reared in traditional religious environments. After all, the term *kosher* is not used biblically in Christian texts or establishments; instead it has been used in food contexts by European Jews, as many dictionary definitions indicate. But ironically, the term is never used in Old Testament food or eating contexts either, even though the word *kosher* is of Hebrew origin.[11] Regardless, so-called kosher food selection and dining principles are deeply rooted in ancient Old Testament law, and they are still meticulously applied in Jewish communities throughout the world to this very day—much like they were thousands of years ago. In stark contrast, both contemporary and traditional expressions of Christianity have had little, if anything, to do with that which is kosher, at least since the term was introduced in dining contexts.

Despite any initial orthodox religious perceptions and connotations, in this book the term *Kosher Christianity* is used in a hopeful sense in this book to describe a new future or potential reality; it does not refer to a dispensational prodigal son. The dichotomy of the term is entirely dependent on how people define or perceive the two words—and how

---

11 Strong's H3787 (כשר), meaning "right" or "acceptable," occurring only in Esther 8:5, Ecclesiastes 10:10, and 11:6.

determined they are to remain committed to their original perceptions and definitions. By no means are the words *kosher* and *Christianity* merged to arbitrarily qualify today's dispensational or yesteryear's traditional religious institutions as 'acceptable' from an Old Testament or Jewish standpoint, even though many institutions bear Christian titles. This is exactly where distinctions must be made; tradition and dogma must be parsed from Christian doctrine. As used in the pages of this book, *Kosher Christianity* refers to a non-dispensational view of the Christian faith and approach to Bible interpretation.

Inspiring a Return to Kosher Christianity

Of course, asking people to investigate the Christian faith from the perspective of *Kosher Christianity* is no trivial matter. Not only is reading an entire book a considerable investment in time, but to expend such effort exploring a radically different perspective, as proposed in *Eat Like Jesus*, may be perceived as a daunting task. It is human nature for people to believe that their preexisting or preconceived notions are correct, and it can be difficult to entertain the possibility of misguidance or deception, lest they feel betrayed by God himself. In this way, personal ego and pride can represent potential barriers to objective investigation. Finally, in surveying an alternate viewpoint, readers might encounter some resistance, being alienated or ostracized for even considering an unconventional view of the New Testament or of the Christian faith. But to *Eat Like Jesus* is not to deny the faith—it is to embrace it with more honesty and enthusiasm.

It is possible that those committed to dispensational theology will suggest that this book attempts to "Judaize" Christian believers and even advocates so-called works-based salvation. To the contrary; those aspiring to earn a guaranteed open-ended ticket to eternal life if they *Eat Like Jesus* will not find their hopes validated in this book. Nevertheless, a failure to *Eat Like Jesus* may well reduce not only a person's quality of life, but their overall life expectancy, thereby hastening the person's arrival at his eternal destiny! After all, carnivorous, scavenging, and cannibalistic animals avoided by Jesus and forbidden by Moses—such as swine and shellfish—exhibit higher decomposition rates, accumulate more toxins, and are higher in pathogens and allergens than are foods derived from kosher sources.

Furthermore, because "zeal without knowledge is not good,"[12] it is reasonable to assert that Bible-believing Christians are in some way obligated to investigate alternate minority views. In fact, the book of Proverbs insists that a person weigh both sides of an argument, such as those represented by *Kosher Christianity*, before rendering a decision.[13] Likewise, John's epistle demands that believers "test the spirits"[14] or the teachings, lest they be misled by isolated dogma or a single point of reference. Of course, intelligent readers understand these principles intuitively, and choose to read books that expand their understanding—not those that merely reinforce whatever they have been previously taught. Academically curious, honest readers understand that knowledge should precede action, lest their zeal be misdirected toward unproductive or destructive ends.

In the end, the motivation for returning to *Kosher Christianity* is a matter of individual decision. Above self-preservation, and apart from health, fear, or guilt, people are also inspired by greater ends, such as obedience and love. Knowing that love is the greatest motivator, and that love makes obedience a joy as opposed to a burden, Jesus himself said, *"If you love me, you will obey what I command."*[15] Love inspires people to emulate those they admire; thus, love should be among the reasons to *EAT LIKE JESUS*.

---

12 Proverbs 19:2

13 Proverbs 18:17 (showing partiality is also forbidden per Leviticus 19:15)

14 1 John 4:1

15 John 14:15

Clearing the Path to Kosher Christianity

Given that the path to *Kosher Christianity* has become obscured by dispensational doctrines and obstructed by deceptive mistranslations, this book is written to empower the reader to digest biblical food texts with kosher reasoning. Because key excerpts of Matthew, Mark, Acts, Romans, Corinthians, and Colossians[16] are dogmatically used to espouse anti-kosher rhetoric, these texts will be examined in their original contexts and languages and compared with Leviticus and Genesis texts, so that a more comprehensive biblical dining theology might be presented. As these texts are examined, this book will reconsider answers to the following questions:

✓ Did Jesus really declare all foods to be clean?
✓ Did Jesus equate Moses' law to human tradition?
✓ Did Peter "get up, kill, and eat" unclean animals after his vision?
✓ Did James recommend fewer commandments for Gentiles?
✓ Did Paul eliminate all Roman and Corinthian eating restrictions?
✓ Did God call Daniel to be a vegetarian?
✓ Did God give Noah permission to eat pigs after the flood?
✓ Did God expect Adam and Eve to eat only vegetables?

However, before Scripture is scrutinized to resolve these stomach-centric questions, the reader is presented with a greater question: *"Is it reasonable to assume that God is good, and that he gave good laws through Moses for the good of man?"*

If a reader is compelled to answer "no" to this question, insinuating that God is ill-intended, there is little hope that the content of this book will be capable of mending such emotional wounds. Subsequent pages are not written to those committed to a prodigal attitude—being determined to remain estranged from the Father, eating among pigs

---

16 Particular texts include Matthew 15:11, 18–20; Mark 7:15, 18–20; Acts 10:15, 11:9; Romans 14:2,14; 1 Corinthians 10:27–31; Colossians 2:20–22

in a distant land. Objecting to the possibility of God's goodness is to remain on a broad superhighway leading to destruction. It is to brand Kosher Christianity as a fallacy without due consideration.

Conversely, readers willing to affirm the goodness of God are those willing to step onto a narrow path, leading to a tree of life. To answer "yes" to the question of God's goodness is to take a leap of faith; it is to "test the spirits" and weigh positions that favor traditional and dispensational dining dogma against scriptural arguments that oppose them. It is to respond openly and impartially to the appeal to *EAT LIKE JESUS*. To answer "yes" is to accept the possibility that *Kosher Christianity* might be the only honorable legacy for the entire family of faith.

1

Jesus, Moses, and the Elders' Traditions

... don't you see that nothing that enters a man from the outside can make him 'unclean'? For it doesn't go into their heart but into their stomach, and then out of the body. (In saying this, Jesus declared all foods "clean.")

—Mark 7:18, 19 NIV

Cleanliness is next to godliness.

—origin uncertain

Cleanliness is next to godliness. At least that's what people used to say—before Western society at large turned sterile, scientific, and secular. However, in recent years, people are no longer conditioned to associate cleanliness with godliness; even among religious audiences, citing this obscure cleanliness-godliness proverb is unlikely to prompt a change in behavior or even elicit a useful response.

Despite its dwindling familiarity, the motto should not be dismissed without due consideration. Instead, it should solicit a number of questions, such as: What meaning might such a proverb convey? Why did the proverb come to be, and why is it no longer popular? Where did it come from? Who first made this claim? When was the saying introduced, and when does it apply? How are cleanliness and godliness really related? Is there significance, either logical or theological, to this proverb?

From Clean Traditions to Clean Technologies

For religious people familiar with Bible texts, it should not be difficult to recall a few of the many Scriptures pertaining to topics of cleanliness and godliness. Yet despite having an ability to recall particular cleanliness-godliness texts, it is unlikely that people will associate such Scriptures with contexts of physical cleansing in everyday situations. Since New Testament canonization, physical cleanliness has generally not been held as something central to church teachings and traditions. As such, religious institutions typically refrain from using the word *clean* in religious affairs, especially in physical contexts.

Even though cleanliness appears to be omitted from religious discussions and excluded from the agendas of religious organizations, it is fortunate that Christians remain compelled to uphold certain cleanliness traditions—such as hand washing—apart from their religious institutions. While hand washing appears to be Pharisaic or Jewish in origin (according to New Testament texts), its usefulness cannot be disputed. After all, it has been scientifically proven that cleanliness was an essential aspect of human health and hygiene long before indoor plumbing made hand washing a custom within reach.

Despite the diminishing religious use of the cleanliness-godliness proverb, many modern technologies are dependent on unprecedented levels of cleanliness as mankind pursues omnipotence and omniscience. Far surpassing the cleanliness standards of the medical industry, 'clean rooms' of microchip and nanotechnology industries have taken *clean* to an entirely new level. In these contexts, *clean* has assumed a new meaning; technology industries can now express *clean* in terms of microns, nanometers, or even parts per trillion.

Similarly, parents today have taken sanitation exercises to the next level. While years ago, tap water and a bar of soap were once deemed sufficient for the pre-dining hand-cleansing ritual, the use of anti-bacterial soaps, sani-wipes, and even alcohol-based liquid gel sanitizers[17] is now the norm. However, it appears that over the course of time, the motivation for cleanliness has transformed from religious duty to scientific enlightenment or even commercial liability.

The Great Debate

Long before microbes were observed under the microscope by the watchful eye of science, Pharisees scrutinized Jesus' disciples as they ate their food with unwashed hands. Jesus defended his disciples' behavior, despite how irreligious or unorthodox the religious experts of the day perceived it to be. Jesus even rebuked the religious personalities who blamed and belittled his students for failing to comply with the custom.

Unfortunately, this single exchange between the Pharisees, the disciples, and Jesus has been used over the course of generations to justify the eradication of physical cleanliness distinctions and principles

---

17 Ingredients such as Triclosan, along with excessive sanitizer use, are cited as being hazardous in a Centers for Disease Control study http://www.livestrong.com/article/121354-health-risks-related-hand-sanitizer/

from the Christian religion. On one hand, the Pharisees seem to be arguing in favor of hand washing and promoting cleanliness-godliness connections; yet on the other hand, Jesus seems to make claims to the contrary. However, a careful review of the dialogue, in the context of other Scriptures, demands a drastically different interpretation.

While the religious debate between Jesus and the Jewish Pharisees[18] is captured in gospels of Matthew[19] and Mark, the Mark account documents the discourse more comprehensively, dedicating almost an entire chapter to the hand washing account. Because the numerous cleanliness, dietary, and spiritual issues cannot be understood without reviewing the full context, the entire gospel of Mark excerpt from the popular New International Version translation is cited below:

> The Pharisees and some of the teachers of the law who had come from Jerusalem gathered around Jesus and saw some of his disciples eating food with hands that were "unclean," that is, unwashed. (The Pharisees and all the Jews do not eat unless they give their hands a ceremonial washing, holding to the tradition of the elders. When they come from the marketplace they do not eat unless they wash. And they observe many other traditions, such as the washing of cups, pitchers and kettles.)

> So the Pharisees and teachers of the law asked Jesus, "Why don't your disciples live according to the tradition of the elders instead of eating their food with unclean hands?"

> He replied, "Isaiah was right when he prophesied about you hypocrites; as it is written:
> 'These people honor me with their lips,
>   but their hearts are far from me.
> They worship me in vain;

---

18 The Pharisaic actions and sentiments in Mark 7 should not be considered as representative of all Jewish and/or Pharisaic thought.
19 Matthew 15:1–11

their teachings are but rules taught by men.'

"You have let go of the commands of God and are holding on to the traditions of men."

And he said to them: "You have a fine way of setting aside the commands of God in order to observe your own traditions! For Moses said, 'Honor your father and your mother,' and, 'Anyone who curses his father or mother must be put to death.' But you say that if a man says to his father or mother: 'Whatever help you might otherwise have received from me is Corban' (that is, a gift devoted to God), then you no longer let him do anything for his father or mother. Thus you nullify the word of God by your tradition that you have handed down. And you do many things like that."

Again Jesus called the crowd to him and said, "Listen to me, everyone, and understand this. Nothing outside a man can make him 'unclean' by going into him. Rather, it is what comes out of a man that makes him 'unclean.'"

After he had left the crowd and entered the house, his disciples asked him about this parable. "Are you so dull?" he asked. "Don't you see that nothing that enters a man from the outside can make him 'unclean'? For it doesn't go into his heart but into his stomach, and then out of his body." (In saying this, Jesus declared all foods "clean.")

He went on: "What comes out of a man is what makes him 'unclean.' For from within, out of men's hearts, come evil thoughts, sexual immorality, theft, murder, adultery, greed, malice, deceit, lewdness, envy, slander, arrogance and folly. All these evils come from inside and make a man 'unclean.'" (Mark 7:1–23 NIV)

Unfortunately, this text, along with the parallel account of Matthew, is illegitimately and frequently used to seed unkosher and lawless philosophies; both passages have been used to nurture antinomian views of the Bible and to negate numerous teachings of Moses.

The popular conclusion, as seemingly emphasized in the contemporary NIV translation above, is that Jesus overturned old commandments of Moses, including so-called kosher laws, in favor of greater 'spiritual' truths and matters of the heart. But while pondering this text, the reader might be compelled to ask, "What is the meaning of this discourse and teaching?" or "Was this account divinely recorded such that all Old Testament cleanliness and food laws could be negated or dismissed?"

Hard Hearts, Hard of Hearing, and Hardly Seeing

In the case of the great debate in the seventh chapter of Mark, Jesus presented what appeared to be a simple teaching to a varied lot of characters. The text implies the audience was diverse, ranging from self-appointed religious experts to curious onlookers to committed disciples. But after delivering his kosher synopsis, Jesus departed, probably leaving much of his audience confused and frustrated—to the point where his close disciples asked for clarification.[20]

Strange as it may seem, Jesus spoke as he did knowing that his parables would not be understood by many. But this should be expected; Jesus revealed to his disciples that not all people would comprehend his teachings. He also indicated that the uniform distribution of knowledge and comprehension was not necessarily his goal. But why?

In different gospel accounts of Jesus' teaching, the disciples had asked him why he spoke in mysterious parables. Jesus responded,

> The knowledge of the secrets of the kingdom of heaven has been given to you, but not to them. Whoever has will be given more, and he will have an abundance. Whoever does

---

20 Mark 7:17

not have, even what he has will be taken from him. (Matt. 13:11–12)

Quoting Isaiah thereafter, Jesus also explained why revelations were given and received disproportionally.

For this people's heart has become calloused; they hardly hear with their ears, and they have closed their eyes. (Matt. 13:15)

In other words, a person's attitude can drastically influence his perception. A hard-hearted man is destined to be hard of hearing as well as virtually and voluntarily blind.

Given Jesus' revelations on parable interpretation in Matthew's gospel, should the reader assume that the great hand washing debate in the seventh chapter of Mark was perceived uniformly among Jesus' diverse audience? Surely, since their eyes and ears were opened at differing levels, it stands to reason that Jesus' listeners received the message with mixed results. For those looking at Mark's account with open eyes, several truths might be deduced. For example:

✓ The principal argument is one of divine authority versus human religious traditions.
✓ The Pharisees prioritized human washing traditions above law given through Moses, thereby encouraging people to usurp or neglect God's law.
✓ The account addresses human washing and cleanliness; it does not discuss types of animals used for food.
✓ The Pharisaic tradition implied that a person might be made evil by ingesting "unclean" matter.

In order to fully substantiate these assertions, a more detailed step-by-step study of Mark's hand washing account has been provided below.

Human Tradition

To underscore the aspects of human religious tradition exposed and discussed in Mark's account, the text begins by setting the tone with an important contextual backdrop. Logically preceding the Pharisees' dialogue and Jesus' teaching, the account begins by outlining human tradition in the first four verses:

> The Pharisees and some of the teachers of the law who had come from Jerusalem gathered around Jesus and saw some of his disciples eating food with hands that were unclean, that is, unwashed. (The Pharisees and all the Jews do not eat unless they give their hands a ceremonial washing, holding to the tradition of the elders. When they come from the marketplace they do not eat unless they wash. And they observe many other traditions, such as the washing of cups, pitchers and kettles.) (Mark 7:1–4)

Beginning with an obvious focus on ceremonial washings, the text introduces the problem and theme of Jewish tradition. This is not to say that all Jewish or human tradition is a problem or unconditionally incorrect, but from these first four verses, the following observations can be made.

- ✓ Unwashed hands were assumed to be unclean hands.
- ✓ The ceremonial washing of hands and dining utensils was considered to be a tradition of the elders.
- ✓ The tradition of the elders governed the behavior of Pharisees and Jews before meals and following marketplace visits.
- ✓ The tradition of the elders was evidently well established; such practices were familiar in Israel, probably for generations.
- ✓ The scope of the traditions of the elders included cleansing of dining implements.

Seeing this information from the first four verses in the proper light is pivotal, since they introduce the central theme of the entire text, and because Jesus' statements are without pertinence if this preamble is not fully understood. After reviewing these first four verses, however, many conclude with closed eyes that the "tradition of the elders" defined cleanliness practices verbatim according to Moses' Old Testament stipulations. However, verses to follow demonstrate the fallacy of such interpretation; Moses' commandments on cleansing and cleanliness are not identical to the practices or "tradition of the elders" as described above.

Continuing Contrasts—Moses versus the Elders

Continuing with Mark's account, the vivid contrast between the religious tradition and the commands of God is succinctly and repeatedly underscored. As in the majority of Jesus' rebukes recorded in the gospel accounts, the basis for argument and dialogue is provided by the Pharisees, who introduce two topics of debate with a single morally loaded question. The account continues,

> So the Pharisees and teachers of the law asked Jesus, 'Why don't your disciples live according to the tradition of the elders instead of eating their food with unclean hands?' He replied, 'Isaiah was right when he prophesied about you hypocrites; as it is written: 'These people honor me with their lips, but their hearts are far from me. They worship me in vain; their teachings are but rules taught by men.' (Mark 7:5–7)

From the religious authorities' own inquiry, it is obvious that they were more concerned about the "tradition of the elders" than they were with Mosaic law. Erring on the side of caution, the religious authorities had presumed the disciples' hands to be unclean; yet circumstance or evidence testifying to the disciples' uncleanness is absent from the text. Furthermore, Jesus' citation of Isaiah would suggest that the

Pharisees' ancient washing traditions were of human origin; as far as true Old Testament commandments were concerned, such traditions were extrapolated at best,[21] and in some cases, altogether impostors. After all, according to Leviticus, eating restrictions were not imposed on "unclean" people apart from festive gatherings,[22] nor had the law stipulated cleansing activities of any sort (e.g., hand washing) prior to the intake of food.

As if quotation of Isaiah's prophecy was inadequate, Jesus again accused the Pharisees, explaining their error to them in his own words. Contrasting God's law with man's law a second time, he rebuked them, saying,

> You have let go of the commands of God and are holding
> on to the traditions of men. (Mark 7:8)

This statement begs two questions: what are the commandments of God and what are the traditions of men? Sadly, many traditional Christian institutions teach congregants to pair one idea with the other; they infer "traditions of men" to mean "laws of Moses." But Jesus never suggested that Mosaic law was to be demoted to that of human invention or pointless ritual; he taught the opposite.[23]

Repetitious Human Traditions

As if the first accusations were insufficient in contrasting Mosaic law with human tradition, Jesus provided yet another example, comparing the Pharisees' behavior against Moses' ideals. Rebuking them, Jesus said,

> You have a fine way of setting aside the commands of God
> in order to observe your own traditions! For Moses said,

---

21 Hand washing traditions might be inferred from Exodus 19:6, 30:19–21; Leviticus 15:11, and Deuteronomy 21:6.

22 Numbers 9:6

23 Matthew 5:17

"Honor your father and your mother," and, "Anyone who curses his father or mother must be put to death." But you say that if a man says to his father or mother: "Whatever help you might otherwise have received from me is Corban" (that is, a gift devoted to God), then you no longer let him do anything for his father or mother. Thus you nullify the word of God by your tradition that you have handed down. And you do many things like that. (Mark 7:9–13)

Since he denounced the religious leaders three times for preferring human traditions over commandments of God declared by Moses, it is no surprise that Jesus would leave the crowd with an accurate account of God's directives pertaining to uncleanness. Again, speaking deliberately and in accordance with Leviticus, Jesus reminded the audience,

Listen to me, everyone, and understand this. Nothing outside a man can make him unclean by going into him. Rather, it is what comes out of a man that makes him unclean. (Mark 7:14–15)

Even though Jesus' earlier statements set clear precedent, as he repeatedly advocates Moses' law above human tradition, the two verses above are nevertheless inferred to teach the very opposite. According to dispensational theologians, these verses are interpreted as Jesus' vocal opposition to Moses' law. But closer examination of the Old Testament Scriptures does not support such this view. In fact, if Jesus' public proclamation is compared with Moses' writings, it becomes evident that Jesus' public teaching was not limited to eating; rather it was a summary of more than a chapter of the book of Leviticus[24] dedicated to hygienic commandments, distilled into just two concise sentences. Jesus was not debunking Moses' cleansing principles; instead, he was succinctly reiterating them.

---

24 Leviticus 5, Leviticus 15, Leviticus 22, Numbers 5

Unclean Sources—Out and On versus In

It is reasonable to deduce from Jesus' words of hygienic wisdom and the Mark 7 introduction that the Pharisees attempted to err on the safe side—even adopting a cleansing philosophy and traditions that were beyond Moses' prescriptions. From Mark 7, it would appear the Pharisees believed that anything unwashed should be regarded as unclean. Likewise, the gospel reader might be vulnerable to making a similar correlation, but only if not familiar with Moses' teachings. After all, Moses never indicated that a person could become unclean by what he ate. To the contrary, Moses indicated that a person could become unclean by that which he touched, and more specifically, by that which his body exuded. In other words, Moses taught that personal uncleanness was contingent on what came *out* of him, or what came *on* to him, but not by what was put *in* to him.

As alluded to in Jesus' concluding statement,[25] personal uncleanness could indeed result from a variety of human bodily discharges. According to Leviticus, discharges such as blood, saliva, phlegm, feces, puss, or semen could render the person with the discharge "unclean," as could rashes or skin disease.[26] Needless to say, all of these bodily fluids are capable of making people unclean, and they would also be regarded as things "coming out of a man," just as Jesus frankly described.

In addition to discharges from the human body, Leviticus also indicates that certain animal varieties were capable of making people unclean. Referring to "unclean" animal varieties, Moses' law explains,

> If a person touches anything ceremonially unclean—whether the carcasses of unclean wild animals or of unclean livestock or of unclean creatures that move along the ground—even though he is unaware of it, he has become unclean and is guilty. (Lev. 5:2)

---

25 Mark 7:15
26 Leviticus 13:14; 15:2, 8; 15:16–19

Note that Moses is not referring to eating as the means by which a person became unclean; instead, he is referring to mere physical and external contact with the carcass. In other words, Moses is referring to a case of *on* and not *in*, even though the very same animal carcasses that were forbidden to eat were also forbidden to touch.

Furthermore, Moses' law included similar provisions for inanimate objects such as utensils and clothing. With similar sanitary concerns, Moses gave instructions relative to unclean animal corpses,

> When one of them dies and falls on something, that article, whatever its use, will be unclean, whether it is made of wood, cloth, hide or sackcloth. Put it in water; it will be unclean till evening, and then it will be clean. (Lev. 11:32)

In all probability, the Pharisaic elders' washing traditions—as applied to hands and utensils—were extrapolated from such commands. However, these Pharisaic directives failed to meet the letter—or the spirit—of Moses' law.

A Crash Course in Levitical Washings

After carefully scrutinizing the washing expectations recorded in Moses' writings, it becomes obvious that people and things subjected to unclean substances would not necessarily attain a status of "clean" if cleansed under the alternate set of washing traditions as introduced by Israel's elders. For example, earthen vessels made of porous clay were not to be treated via ceremonial rinsing if exposed to uncleanness; they were to be destroyed instead.[27] Depending on material of construction, certain objects that were exposed to unclean things were not to be merely rinsed with water; some were to be purified or sterilized by fire.[28] Furthermore, it appears that the elders' tradition as described in Mark 7 failed to incorporate time delays as Moses' cleansing directives required.

---

27 Leviticus 6:28
28 Leviticus 13:55, Numbers 31:23

As for unclean persons, if there was any washing to be done, it was to be done as stipulated by Moses' law. Contrary to the elders' limited hand washing traditions as described in Mark 7, Moses' law instructed,

> Whoever touches the man who has a discharge must wash his clothes and bathe with water, and he will be unclean till evening. (Lev. 15:7)

However obscure or arbitrary the contemporary Gentile Christian may perceive this Mosaic law to be, it is essential to note how Mark's account presents the Pharisees' hand washing effort as superficial in terms of compliance with the Leviticus text.[29] In addition to failing to wait the prescribed time to declare an object or person clean, the Pharisaic tradition also failed to honor the full body wash expectation as established in Moses' writings.

Ironically, according to Leviticus, hand washing was required to be performed by the unclean person with the bodily discharge. Referring to unclean persons, Moses wrote,

> Anyone the man with a discharge touches without rinsing his hands with water must wash his clothes and bathe with water, and he will be unclean till evening. (Lev. 15:11)

In a sense, by washing their own hands, the Pharisees were acting as if they themselves were the unclean persons, who would be technically unfit to attend public dining assemblies without a full body wash. To add to the irony, they were calling the disciples unclean without having a basis for doing so. The Pharisees did not honor the fact that not everything washed per their tradition was clean according to Moses, nor did they seem to accept the possibility that something could be

---

29 A precautionary washing request or tradition in accordance with Leviticus 15:11 is not unreasonable as a matter of habit or prudence, but should not be interpreted as a standing mandate either. Eating while in an unclean state was still permitted (ref. Deuteronomy 12:15), provided that contact with others or communal food (e.g., Deuteronomy 26:14) was avoided.

clean even though it was not washed.[30] Instead, they zealously presumed every person, place, and thing was dirty;[31] they meticulously washed only implements and extremities as a precaution; and they incorrectly surmised that their washing rituals immediately cleaned everything. However, contrary to the elders' expectations, Moses did nothing to prohibit an unclean man from eating or from handling his own food while he was in an unclean state.

Unclean and Evil Origins

Through manmade religious washing rituals, the Pharisaic sects had deceived the people into believing they might be made unclean as a result of incidental ingestion of minuscule unclean or defiled matter— as if it might permeate the stomach and overcome the spirit or 'heart' of a man, compromising his moral fortitude. The people came to mistake the elders' rituals for Moses' mandates. They accepted Pharisaic paranoia in place of Moses' prudence. Thus, Jesus was compelled to reiterate Moses' teachings relative to the topic of cleanliness, setting the record straight before the Pharisees.

However, Jesus did not elaborate on the moral implications of his two-sentence synopsis of Leviticus until he withdrew from the crowd, and until after his disciples inquired of him. Mark also records this private inquiry, in which the spiritual aspects of the Pharisees' doctrinal error become more obvious.

> After he had left the crowd and entered the house, his disciples asked him about this parable. "Are you so dull?" he asked. "Don't you see that nothing that enters a man from the outside can make him 'unclean'? For it doesn't go into his heart but into his stomach, and then out of his body." (In saying this, Jesus declared all foods "clean.")

---

30 Grain collected directly from a field was not considered unclean, e.g., Matthew 12:1.

31 Mark 7:1-4

> He went on: "What comes out of a man is what makes him
> 'unclean.' For from within, out of men's hearts, come evil
> thoughts, sexual immorality, theft, murder, adultery, greed,
> malice, deceit, lewdness, envy, slander, arrogance and folly.
> All these evils come from inside and make a man 'unclean.'"
> (Mark 7:17–23)

Unfortunately, in interpreting these isolated gospel texts without Moses' law, many people infer Jesus' private remarks to be outright permission to ignore the physical mandates in favor of the spiritual revelation, not taking into account the illegitimate Pharisaic cause-effect theology that Jesus was dispelling.

Jesus had to clarify to his disciples that evil or immoral behavior was not the consequence of eating dirty food. It stands to reason that Jesus did not make this statement in a vacuum. To the contrary, he had to underscore where evil came from because the traditions and teachings of the religious authorities were so pervasive, confounding, and effective in distorting the truth pertaining to the origin of evil. From the account, there is every reason to believe that Pharisaic behavior had led the disciples—and the masses—to believe that evil or evil inclinations could manifest within people because of something they ingested orally. They took the old "you are what you eat" adage a step too far, inferring that a person who ate evil would become evil!

If not for the prevailing perceptions on the external origin of evil inclinations, Jesus' closing comments in Mark 7 must be viewed as an abrupt change of subject and a topic out of context, especially if Levitical teachings are not considered. However, in acknowledging the simple truth of Leviticus in its entirety—namely, "that what comes out of a man makes him unclean"—Jesus' private revelations following the debate must be interpreted as supplementary information, as opposed to statements overturning or correcting previous Mosaic instructions. To reiterate, *Jesus never challenged relationships between physical illness and unclean animal varieties used for food; instead, he underscored the disconnect between physically dirty hands and moral depravity.* As such, Jesus' teachings were a far cry from declaring all foods to be "clean."

Liberal Interpretation of Literal Writing

Nevertheless, out of unfamiliarity with—or possibly in contempt of—Moses' law, some take Jesus' concluding remarks to illogical extremes, distorting his words to negate not only elementary hygiene laws, but extending even greater distortions to the dietary laws. Many English Bible translations liberally state outright that "Jesus declared all foods clean." However, in examining many older English translations, [32] it becomes apparent that most texts exclude the misleading parenthetical statement from verse 19 ("Jesus declared all foods clean"). For example, the Shakespearean King James Version interprets the text,

> "And he saith unto them, Are ye so without understanding also? Do ye not perceive, that whatsoever thing from without entereth into the man, it cannot defile him; because it entereth not into his heart, but into the belly, and goeth out into the draught, purging all meats? And he said, That which cometh out of the man, that defileth the man." (Mark 7:18–20 KJV)

In comparing this old English with more contemporary translations, as demonstrated on page 15-16, it becomes apparent that Jesus' parenthetical food cleansing claim is completely absent from the King James text. Likewise, a word-for-word interlinear translation[33] is more consistent with the King James text, leaving a gaping hole where the New International Version adds the ambitious claim that Jesus "declared all foods clean." To illustrate this, the Greek-English interlinear translation[34] of Mark 7:19-20 is provided below.

---

32 An extensive listing of additional Mark 7:19 English translations, along with further translation assessments, have been included in chapter 5 for ease of comparison.
33 Interlinear Greek text is based upon Textus Receptus.
34 From Interlinear Scripture Analyzer (ISA) software per www.scripture4all.org.

7:19 ΟΤΙ ΟΥΚ ΕΙCΠΟΡΕΥΕΤΑΙ ΑΥΤΟΥ ΕΙC

hoti ou eisporeuomai autos eis

Conj Part Neg vi Pres midD/pasD 3 Sg pp Gen Sg m Prep

that NOT it-IS-INTO-GOING OF-him INTO
it-is-going-in

ΤΗΝ ΚΑΡΔΙΑΝ ΑΛΛ ΕΙC ΤΗΝ ΚΟΙΛΙΑΝ

ho kardia alla eis ho koilia

t_ Acc Sg f n_ Acc Sg f Conj Prep t_ Acc Sg f n_ Acc Sg f

THE HEART but INTO THE CAVITY
bowel

ΚΑΙ ΕΙC ΤΟΝ ΑΦΕΔΡΩΝΑ ΕΚΠΟΡΕΥΕΤΑΙ

kai eis ho aphedrOn ekporeuomai

Conj Prep t_ Acc Sg m n_ Acc Sg m vi Pres midD/pasD 3 Sg

AND INTO THE FROM-SETTLE it-IS-OUT-GOING
latrine it-is-going-out

ΚΑΘΑΡΙΖΩΝ ΠΑΝΤΑ ΤΑ ΒΡΩΜΑΤΑ

katharizO pas ho brOma

vp Pres Act Nom Sg m a_ Acc Pl n t_ Acc Pl n n_ Acc Pl n

cleansING ALL THE FOODS

7:20 ΕΛΕΓΕΝ ΔΕ ΟΤΙ ΤΟ ΕΚ ΤΟΥ

legO de hoti ho ek ho

vi impf Act 3 Sg Conj Conj t_ Nom Sg n Prep t_ Gen Sg m

He-said YET that THE OUT OF-THE

ΑΝΘΡΩΠΟΥ ΕΚΠΟΡΕΥΟΜΕΝΟΝ ΕΚΕΙΝΟ

anthrOpos ekporeuomai ekeinos

n_ Gen Sg m vp Pres midD/pasD Nom Sg n pd Nom Sg n

human OUT-GOING that
going-out

ΚΟΙΝΟΙ ΤΟΝ ΑΝΘΡΩΠΟΝ

koinoO ho anthrOpos

vi Pres Act 3 Sg t_ Acc Sg m n_ Acc Sg m

IS-COMMONING THE human
is-contaminating

From the Greek text above, it is clear that the original language fails to support the parenthetical "Jesus declared all foods clean" statement. However, if the text is rendered without superfluous interjection, Jesus' teaching is better understood and is not twisted to mislead the reader. The Greek text describes the passage of food through the body, where food goes from field to hand to market to hand to mouth to stomach to latrine, with stomach acid and the bowels processing whatever a person might have ingested accidentally. It is credible to reason that Jesus described the digestive process as one of cleansing, the stomach acid compensating for minor contaminants that a person might ingest due to contact with unwashed hands. But the digestive process would not leave the matter "clean" in the latrine in the end, as human defecation (regardless of preceding diet or preparation of food) is cited as uncleanness by Moses and the prophet Ezekiel alike.[35] Instead, the bowels were what was being "cleansed" or "purged" or "flushed." Thus, Jesus' point in the gospel of Mark was simple: whatever you eat will be expelled from the body, and nothing evil will rub off on you on the inside as it passes through your system!

Common English and Unclean Greek

Adding to the confusion, words resembling "unclean" are not translated consistently in English Bible translations. In fact, "unclean" and other words including "defile," "defiled," "foul," "polluted," "unholy," and "common" are used somewhat interchangeably in the place of three different Greek words, which also carry unique and distinct connotations.

For example, the Greek word in Mark chapter 7 describing the disciples' unwashed hands (κοινός/koinos)[36] is an adjective that might be most universally translated as "common" or "shared," as it can always

---

35 Deuteronomy 23:12, Ezekiel 4:12–15
36 Strong's G2839, e.g., Mark 7:2

be related to public or community contexts.[37] Yet even though κοινός/koinos occurs in New Testament texts outside of cleanliness or moral contexts,[38] the translators—much like the Pharisees—nevertheless opted to interpret the terms with negative connotations in particular places, using words like "defiled" or "unclean" to describe the disciples' hands. As suggested previously, the actual state of the disciples' hands prior to their encounter with the Pharisees is uncertain. Therefore, it stands to reason that, where used biblically in various New Testament contexts, the English adjective "unclean" would be better understood as something "un-clean;" that is, something of *uncertain* purity or cleanliness, as opposed to something that is positively identified to be dirty or defiled. For such reasons, a more accurate and morally neutral term, such as "common," should be considered for all New Testament occurrences of κοινός/koinos, lest the reader be coaxed into drawing presumptive conclusions.

Moreover, it is of note that the adjective κοινός/koinos is only attributed to objects, and that these "common" or "shared" objects are not credited with the unconditional ability to "defile" or "make unclean," as translators also suggest when interpreting the Greek verb κοινόω/koinoō[39]. In further emphasizing communal connotations and links between κοινός/koinos and κοινόω/koinoō, it becomes evident that Jesus' use of the verb κοινόω/koinoō in the Mark 7 account has more to do with "making common" and less to do with corrupting or polluting. Of course, by implication, the verb κοινόω/koinoō strongly implies to "make unholy," as the term "holy" refers to something that is "set apart," which is the very opposite of something that is "common," "shared," or "public." Therefore, it would be appropriate to suggest that Jesus said that nothing "common" (κοινός/koinos) is capable of "commoning" (κοινόω/koinoō), i.e., *making* people "common" or "unholy." Thus, the New Testament indicates that people are not to be

---

37 Strong's G2842 (κοινωνία/koinōnia), meaning fellowship or community, likely correlates to Strong's G2862 (κολωνία/kolōnia), meaning colony.
38 Acts 2:44, Acts 4:32, Titus 1:4, Jude 1:3
39 Strong's G2840

described as *common* (κοινός/koinos),[40] and that people could not be *made unholy* (κοινόω/koinoō) spiritually from encountering something that is common.

The Mark 7 account, however, makes no reference to the Greek adjectives that may be used to describe food of an unclean variety, such as meat derived from the types of animals that Moses forbade to eat. Derived from a different word, the adjective ακαθαρτος (akathartos, which is an antonym for clean)[41] is used to describe evil spirits and animals of an unredeemable variety—having the power to corrupt— which Jesus never cleansed. Although Jesus cleansed people of spirits and ailments which were ακαθαρτος (akathartos) by nature, he never cleansed animals or foods that were ακαθαρτος (akathartos). Things such as mold, parasites, or evil spirits would be described as ακαθαρτος (akathartos), in the same way that the Bible describes unclean animals such as pigs, shellfish and cockroaches. Essentially, the Pharisees of Mark 7 ascribed the same attributes of unclean things, which are ακαθαρτος (akathartos), to all things common (κοινός/koinos).

Spiritually Unclean Food and Proper Repentance

While Jesus did say that ingesting mishandled or "common" things would not render a man evil, it is of critical importance to reiterate that the surrounding or parallel accounts make no mention of various animal/food types and their Old Testament distinctions. Making a theological commitment to dispensational dogma, common English and unclean Greek interpretations, or superfluous translations will ultimately pervert, not to mention invert, the gospel message. Instead of promising forgiveness in response to repentance, the substitute gospel becomes, "Jesus died—Moses' dietary and cleanliness laws need not apply!"

This message of lawlessness is the polar opposite of the true gospel,

---

40 Acts 10:28

41 Strong's G2511 (καθαρίζω/katharizō) in verbal form a means "cleaning" or "purging." Strong's G2513 (καθαρισμός/katharismos) as an adjective means "clean."

particularly as it appears in conjunction with some of Jesus' earliest recorded teachings. For example, according to Matthew, the mandate of repentance is inseparable from the gospel or "good news" idea.

> After John was put in prison, Jesus went into Galilee, proclaiming the good news of God. 'The time has come,' he said. 'The kingdom of God is near. Repent and believe the good news!' (Matt. 11:25–26).

Whether in English, Hebrew, or Greek, the words for *repent*[42] carry connotations beyond regret; they always imply change and return. But without a standard whereby morality is determined, the idea of repentance is almost pointless—it is speculative at best. True repentance requires an affirmative standard by which to define good deeds, just as it requires a prohibitive standard or commandments in order to define deviant behavior.

Thus, repentance without Moses' standards for reference is folly; it is arbitrary and baseless. The same repentance-gospel relationship was conveyed by John the Baptist before he was imprisoned.[43] It defies logic to propose that John and Jesus were attempting to preach a new form of repentance or to convince the children of Israel to 'return' to a new gospel. While theologians imply that the gospel message is limited to teachings in the era of Jesus' incarnation, every book of the Bible points to the fact that the gospel is timeless: there is no time like the present to repent from evil and be restored to the Creator.

Mark's Message

Despite the way those claiming to represent Christian institutions and doctrines may try to represent the teachings of Jesus, a simple truth cannot be overstated: Jesus never made any attempt to redefine

---

42 "תשובה"or "teshuvah" in Hebrew, Strong's H8666
43 Luke 3:7–18

either food[44] or cleanliness as stipulated by Moses. He did not compel his disciples to adopt behaviors contrary to those of Moses, as did the Pharisees of the gospel accounts. Regardless of calendar date, BC or AD, God's Word conveyed through Moses, along with the definition of *repentance*, remains unchanged. To paraphrase Mark, Matthew, Moses, and Jesus, what comes out of people can make them unclean, but eating common or dirty food won't make people evil!

---

44 Matthew 7:10 implies that a snake (an unclean animal) is an unsuitable substitute for a fish.

Chapter 1 Notes

2

Peter's Vision and Gentile Dining Acts

Then a voice told him, "Get up, Peter. Kill and eat."

"Surely not, Lord!" Peter replied. "I have never eaten anything impure or unclean."

The voice spoke to him a second time, "Do not call anything impure that God has made clean."

—Acts 10:13–15

Usually presented in concert with mistranslated and out of context citations of the seventh chapter of Mark, there are other popular New Testament texts that appear to relinquish Moses' dietary laws for all of Christendom. For example, in the book of Acts, there is a short story where Peter seems to receive permission from Heaven itself to embrace an unkosher omnivore diet. Extracted from its greater context, Peter's remarkable animal vision is presented below.

> About noon the following day as they were on their journey and approaching the city, Peter went up on the roof to pray. He became hungry and wanted something to eat, and while the meal was being prepared, he fell into a trance.
>
> He saw heaven opened and something like a large sheet being let down to earth by its four corners. It contained all kinds of four-footed animals, as well as reptiles of the earth and birds of the air.
>
> Then a voice told him, "Get up, Peter. Kill and eat."
>
> "Surely not, Lord!" Peter replied. "I have never eaten anything impure or unclean."
>
> The voice spoke to him a second time, "Do not call anything impure that God has made clean."
>
> This happened three times, and immediately the sheet was taken back to heaven. (Acts 10:9–16)

After reading Peter's "kill and eat!" vision recorded in the tenth chapter of Acts, it is obvious that the account makes references to Old Covenant dietary regulations. In fact, Acts 10 even makes direct reference to animal types used for food—unlike the Mark 7 dialogue, which instead discussed topics of mealtime cleansing traditions and the origin of evil.

Regardless, it is without due consideration of the greater New Testament contexts that this text is often interpreted as unkosher reinforcement of Mark 7; it is assumed to reiterate the idea that "Jesus made all animals clean." After all, Peter was instructed to "kill and eat" right after he saw a sheet containing various animals descending from heaven. Additionally, a voice from heaven commanded Peter, "Do not call anything impure that God has made clean." According to traditional teachings, these texts prove beyond a reasonable doubt that the New Testament permits Christian disciples to eat anything and everything.

Clean Precedent

Peter, however, responded to the contrary, emphatically testifying to his individual commitment to Moses' law. But why was Peter so stubborn and compelled to object—even after hearing a voice from heaven three times? Why didn't he give in and agree to the heavenly request at some point?

Given the circumstances, it is prudent to first evaluate Peter's protests from the perspective of precedent, in that he boasted a perfect record of upholding Moses' dietary law. While the response "I have never eaten anything unclean" bears striking resemblance to the words of the prophet Ezekiel uttered centuries prior,[45] the use of precedent is really more applicable to Peter's experiences within his own lifetime. Curiously enough, despite all of Peter's character flaws and shortcomings, which are candidly disclosed in New Testament texts, the gospel texts never offer any information to undermine Peter's claims to kosher compliance. After all, Peter could have easily fished shellfish and catfish out of the

---

45 Per Ezekiel 4:14, the prophet Ezekiel objected to cooking his food over human excrement during unusual prophetic circumstances, insisting that he had never eaten anything unclean.

Sea of Galilee; and as a professional fisherman and miracle witness, Peter could have even fished for pork out of the same lake subsequent to Jesus' exorcism of a legion of demons, which resulted in a mass swine drowning![46] Nevertheless, the voice from heaven neither faulted Peter for failure to comply with Moses' dietary law, nor rebuked him for boasting without basis. In other words, after Peter's claim to dietary perfection, the heavenly voice did not tell Peter, "That's impossible, Peter! Moses' food laws are too hard for you to keep."

Peter's precedent demands a simple answer to a simple question; "If Jesus 'declared all foods clean,' why did Peter refuse to accept this earlier teaching of Jesus?" For had Jesus declared all foods clean in Mark 7, then Peter would have responded differently in his vision, only claiming that he never ate anything unclean before Jesus told him that he could do otherwise.

This problem of the unclean-animals-for-food precedent clearly extends into earlier gospel teachings and narratives as well. Given that the Acts account is the first of the New Testament to allude to the ingestion of unclean animal varieties, it is most curious that Jesus did nothing to notify his audience of the pending or upcoming change to the law—either by authoritative declaration, by public consent, by public example, or by prophetic prediction. Why would Jesus defer such important and potentially controversial changes to God's law through Moses until after his ascension? It's not as if Jesus had a reputation for retreating from controversy; he didn't abandon debates, cowering in fear. Why wouldn't Jesus personally take a more direct approach, a stronger stance on recanting Moses' dietary law, leaving it recorded for all in gospel texts? Why introduce such a radical food law paradigm shift through a single man without witnesses, and why leave such a critical matter up to a brief set of enigmatic visions?

Not only is the lack of unkosher precedent relevant to Jesus' teaching and Peter's visionary claims, but it also applies to every one of Jesus' disciples. Not a single one of the twelve is described in New Testament texts as indulging in an unkosher diet. Moreover, the animals in Peter's

---

46 Mark 5:11

vision were imaginary; and there is no evidence that he satisfied his appetite in accordance with the vision on awakening. In fact, the account fails to describe Peter's post-vision lunchtime cuisine, and the text remains silent with respect to Peter's future dietary habits.

Peter, Linnaeus, and Moses

Instead of guessing about Peter's diet and speculating as to why he did not concede in his vision, perhaps it would be prudent to first consider exactly what Peter saw. Referring to the sheet in Peter's vision, the Acts text describes,

> Wherein were all manner of fourfooted beasts of the earth, and wild beasts, and creeping things, and fowls of the air. (Acts 10:12—KJV)

While the Acts listing of quadrupeds, wild beasts, creeping things, and flying things may sound vague by today's elaborate Latin-based animal taxonomy systems, it is of note that these animal groups correspond with earlier biblical animal classifications. Long before Carl Linnaeus and his system of animal classification was conceived, God had established one through Moses—and Peter was undoubtedly familiar with it.

Moses' system was not scientifically complex, dividing organisms into species from genus, families, orders, classes, phylum, kingdoms, and domains as Linnaeus did. Moses' system of animal classification employed two primary categories: clean and unclean. By means of these two principal classifications, God described what people could and could not eat—as well as what they could and should not touch. Other than the clean and unclean, Moses referred to only four simple animal classifications or subcategories: land-dwellers, aquatic creatures, flying things, and crawling things, as depicted on the book cover.

Among the four principal animal subcategories, the distinctions between clean and unclean were simple, and are delineated by the writings of Moses cited below.

> Of all the animals that live on land, these are the ones you may eat: You may eat any animal that has a split hoof completely divided and that chews the cud. There are some that only chew the cud or only have a split hoof, but you must not eat them. (Lev. 11:2–4)

> Of all the creatures living in the water of the seas and the streams, you may eat any that have fins and scales. But all creatures in the seas or streams that do not have fins and scales—whether among all the swarming things or among all the other living creatures in the water—you are to detest. And since you are to detest them, you must not eat their meat and you must detest their carcasses. Anything living in the water that does not have fins and scales is to be detestable to you. (Lev. 11:9–12)

> These are the birds you are to detest and not eat because they are detestable: the eagle, the vulture, the black vulture, the red kite, any kind of black kite, any kind of raven, the horned owl, the screech owl, the gull, any kind of hawk, the little owl, the cormorant, the great owl, the white owl, the desert owl, the osprey, the stork, any kind of heron, the hoopoe and the bat. (Lev. 11:13–19)

> All flying insects that walk on all fours are to be detestable to you. There are, however, some winged creatures that walk on all fours that you may eat: those that have jointed legs for hopping on the ground. Of these you may eat any kind of locust, katydid, cricket or grasshopper. But all other winged creatures that have four legs you are to detest. (Lev. 11:20–23)

Although the New Testament is by no means a book created to extensively describe animal anatomy and taxonomy, it is interesting that the animals of Peter's Acts vision correlate perfectly with the main

Levitical subcategories,[47] with the exception of aquatic creatures, which were excluded from the vision. It stands to reason, then, that among the types of animals Peter saw, there were two kinds—clean[48] and unclean.[49]

Peter, however, rejected the entire lot of animals outright. Yet Peter's problem was not in rejecting unclean animals as food, but rather in rejecting all animals—the clean animals along with the unclean ones. In other words, Peter pronounced all of the clean animal varieties to be "common" (κοινός/koinos)[50] based upon their proximity to unclean animals, and therefore inedible, given that they were corralled with the unclean (ακάθαρτος/akathartos)[51] ones. But the voice from heaven did not rebuke Peter for refusing to eat the animals that were unclean (or ακάθαρτος/ akathartos); instead, the voice warned Peter about making things to be common or unholy (κοινόω/koinoō).[52] He made blanket statements about the animals; his problems were therefore those of discernment and separation. Peter protested, "Surely not!" when he probably should have responded, "Kill and eat what?" since there would also have been clean varieties on the white sheet menu from which he could choose. [53]

Peter's Puzzle

In trying to comprehend Peter's vision, it is also important to consider things from Peter's perspective. For example, what did Peter think the "Get up, kill, and eat" vision meant? Did he interpret his

---

47 Levitical categories also correspond with groups defined in Genesis 1.

48 The Greek phrase, "πάντα τὰ τετράποδα τῆς γῆς" used in Acts 10:12 refers to all (Strong's G3956) quadrupeds, which includes clean animal varieties per Leviticus 11.

49 The Greek terms used to describe "wild beasts" and "crawling things" (Strong's G2342 and G2062) refer to unclean animal varieties per Leviticus 11.

50 Strong's G2839

51 Strong's G169

52 The original Greek verb (Strong's G2840) implies that Peter was not merely calling clean things common, but making them common.

53 It is possible that Peter, seeking to avoid fecal contamination from unclean animals, would not eat clean animals corralled in close proximity with unclean animals.

vision as "Go ahead and eat the unclean animals," or did he understand the instruction and vision in some other way?

Apparently, during the vision, Peter was praying on a rooftop. If the "rise-kill-eat" commandment was meant to be fulfilled literally, surely it would require some sort of living unclean animal to be present with him on the roof. However, in examining the Acts chapter 10 and 11 accounts, it is reasonable to infer that lunch was being prepared for Peter. Thus, when Peter did get up from his prayer-trance-vision, he was not literally inclined to kill, since a meal was being prepared for him. Neither was Peter's first post-vision response to eat, nor is there evidence that Peter was being served something unclean. Peter was clearly puzzled at the conclusion of the vision, and he continued to ponder what he had experienced, trying desperately to understand.

Of course, Peter's saga did not conclude with him dwelling on the "kill and eat" mandate. Thus the plot thickens as the Acts account continues,

> While Peter was still thinking about the vision, the Spirit said to him, "Simon, three men are looking for you. So get up and go downstairs. Do not hesitate to go with them, for I have sent them." (Acts 10:19–20)

Obviously, "kill and eat" would not be a prudent way to receive divinely dispatched houseguests; hence Peter did not respond by murder and cannibalism following the knock at the door.

Peter's Missing Puzzle Pieces

After greeting his guests, the Acts account records additional details of Peter's divine appointments following his vision. A devout Roman centurion named Cornelius, who had a complementary vision, had sent three of his men to summon Peter to Caesarea. During his road trip with the men between Joppa and Caesarea, Peter had time to ponder the circumstances—past, present, and future—in light of his curious "kill and eat" vision. The meaning of his vision would not be fully revealed until he arrived at his destination, at the behest of the centurion. Explaining his assorted-animal "kill and eat" vision, Peter's story and testimony continue.

> Talking with him, Peter went inside and found a large gathering of people. He said to them: "You are well aware that it is against our law for a Jew to associate with a Gentile or visit him. But God has shown me that I should not call any man impure or unclean. So when I was sent for, I came without raising any objection. May I ask why you sent for me?
>
> Cornelius answered: "Four days ago I was in my house praying at this hour, at three in the afternoon. Suddenly a man in shining clothes stood before me and said, 'Cornelius, God has heard your prayer and remembered your gifts to the poor. Send to Joppa for Simon who is called Peter. He is a guest in the home of Simon the tanner, who lives by the sea.' So I sent for you immediately, and it was good of you to come. Now we are all here in the presence of God to listen to everything the Lord has commanded you to tell us.'
>
> Then Peter began to speak: "I now realize how true it is that God does not show favoritism but accepts men from every nation who fear him and do what is right."
>
> … while Peter was still speaking these words, the Holy Spirit came on all who heard the message. The circumcised believers who had come with Peter were astonished that the gift of the Holy Spirit had been poured out even on the Gentiles. For they heard them speaking in tongues and praising God. (Acts 10:27–35, 44–46)

Alas, the interpretation of Peter's "kill and eat" vision is unveiled— completely devoid of food types, dining habits, cleansing rituals, or culinary contexts! Just as his vision indicated, Peter was in the habit of categorically rejecting the Gentiles as "unholy" or "common," regardless of whether they were clean or unclean. Peter assumes no eating connections from his earlier vision; instead, his self-realization following Cornelius' revelation dealt with his own people perception problems!

Not long after his own personal breakthrough, Peter encountered the same religious bigotry among circumcised believers in Jerusalem, who claimed that his behavior was contrary to their religious tradition.[54] In response, Peter again confessed his own prejudice against Gentiles, citing his "kill and eat" vision in its entirety to teach these believers the error of undue favoritism.[55] On both occasions, Peter recalled the same vision and interpreted it in the same way. Unlike God, Peter and circumcised believers in Jerusalem did not openly accept men from every nation who did what was right. Instead, they isolated themselves from all Gentiles, and rejected the Gentiles as unholy or common.

Jewish Law versus Moses' Law

In his confession, Peter makes a point to differentiate between "our law" (i.e., Jewish law or tradition) and God's law in Acts chapters 10 and 11. In this Acts text, Peter distinguishes between the "two laws" exactly as Jesus had done repeatedly in Mark chapter 7. In Mark's gospel, Jesus suggested that particular Jewish teaching and tradition was not originating from or in agreement with Moses' law; he also provided clarification in saying that eating something unclean could not make you corrupt or evil. In the same way, the Jewish law that polarized Peter and his Jerusalem counterparts into isolating themselves from the uncircumcised Gentiles could not be found in Moses' scrolls.

Although national or ethnic isolation during mealtime was not a Mosaic decree, it is likely that the Jewish tradition of that time was extrapolated from divine commandments given at the time of the

---

54 Acts 11:2–3
55 Acts 11:1–18

Egyptian exodus. In addition to legitimate prohibitions on intermarriage to certain tribes characterized by inbreeding,[56] Moses' Torah did indeed include special and limited social barriers between the circumcised and uncircumcised. Yet these barriers were imposed only for Passover, as described below.

> The Lord said to Moses and Aaron, "These are the regulations for the Passover: No foreigner is to eat of it. Any slave you have bought may eat of it after you have circumcised him, but a temporary resident and a hired worker may not eat of it … An alien living among you who wants to celebrate the Lord's Passover must have all the males in his household circumcised; then he may take part like one born in the land. No uncircumcised male may eat of it. The same law applies to the native-born and to the alien living among you." (Ex. 12:43–45, 48–49)

In Acts, through Peter's vision, God changes no food law, but instead clarifies his expectations for human relations. In the same way that the Pharisees and the teachers of the law had exaggerated and distorted the cleanliness and dietary laws, so too were Peter and his fellow Jews in Jerusalem conditioned to exaggerate the Jews' unique distinction far beyond its God-given Mosaic or prophetic contexts. As made evident by Jesus' teachings in Mark, people were defiled not by what they ate, but by what they exuded or touched, just as indicated in Leviticus. Also, as Peter was reminded in the Acts account, uncleanness[57] was not categorically ascribed to uncircumcised Gentiles; Leviticus implies that Jew and Gentile alike are born unclean.[58] Thereafter, their state

---

56 Deuteronomy 7:1–3 and 22:2–3 prohibit intermarriage with nations originating from inbred or forbidden relationships, ref. Genesis 9:18, 22, 25; Genesis 19:36–38; Leviticus 18:6–8.

57 Strong's G169, ακαθαρτος (akathartos), "impure" or "unclean." The same term is used to describe evil spirits throughout the New Testament, but never people.

58 Leviticus 12 uses Strong's H2930, טמא (ṭâmê'), to describe those contaminated with blood or bodily fluids.

of physical cleanliness would be directly coupled to their adherence to Moses' law, not to their heritage. Moses' law did not forbid an Israelite to eat or associate with his fellow man; this was likely a Jewish extrapolation,[59] perhaps a 'fence law' Pharisaic in origin and intended to protect people from violating kosher commandments, or even intermarrying with nations descended from incestuous relationships.

To the contrary, the law of Moses demanded that the people of Israel welcome the alien with compassion, respect, and justice,[60] just as Abraham welcomed complete strangers[61] several generations before Moses' birth. As a matter of fact, Moses' Torah required Israelite landowners to allow aliens to glean from their fields and vineyards.[62] So, given the circumstances, Peter's interpretation of his "kill and eat" vision should not have been a surprise to either Jewish or other believers who were advocates of Moses' writings.

Spiritual Bigotry and Theological Absurdity

Just in case Peter's personal revelations and the spiritual outpouring would be deemed as an insufficient explanation for his vision, the context of the story of Cornelius is extracted from a larger whole. Following Peter's "kill and eat" vision, Acts expounds even further on theology prevalent within the first century Judeo-Christian community.

According to the Acts account, some men from Jerusalem that were sent to Antioch were confused by the meaning of the covenants of Abraham and Moses, and were teaching,

> Unless you are circumcised, according to the custom taught by Moses, you cannot be saved. (Acts 15:1)

---

59 Possibly from Deuteronomy 26:14
60 Leviticus 19:33–34
61 Genesis 18:2–5
62 Leviticus 19:10

Moreover, Christian believers of Jerusalem, who affiliated with a party of Pharisees, sided with those from Antioch and also insisted,

> The Gentiles must be circumcised and required to obey the law of Moses. (Acts 15:5)

In the ancient covenants, however, neither Abraham nor Moses promised eternal salvation as a result of circumcision, as the Pharisees had insisted; neither was circumcision prescribed for Gentiles outside of Abraham's household. As such, without negating the covenant, the laws of Moses, or the commandment of circumcision, Peter made a point to testify on the Gentiles' behalf and clarify the relationship between circumcision and salvation.

> Brothers, you know that some time ago God made a choice among you that the Gentiles might hear from my lips the message of the gospel and believe. God, who knows the heart, showed that he accepted them by giving the Holy Spirit to them, just as he did to us. He made no distinction between us and them, for he purified their hearts by faith. Now then, why do you try to test God by putting on the necks of the disciples a yoke that neither we nor our fathers have been able to bear? No! We believe it is through the grace of our Lord Jesus that we are saved, just as they are. (Acts 15:7–11)

Clearly, the yoke to which Peter alluded could be described as extra-biblical requirements, which implied salvation was works-based. As they were teaching in Antioch, the Pharisees of Christian affiliation obviously ascribed salvation or redemption to circumcision; moreover, they taught that the Gentiles were required to obey all of Moses' law to be saved. Furthermore, according to Moses, circumcision was to be performed on the eighth day.[63] The Pharisees may have implied

---

63 Leviticus 12:3

that those who missed out on this religious rite and commandment were forever excluded from salvation and the 'chosen people' club. As commanded by Moses, however, this custom was an involuntary endeavor, dictated by heritage and parental decision. The Pharisees visiting Antioch were stretching the texts, implying that salvation was accomplished—in part— through the hands of men, and connecting the covenant and rite to a promise without a basis for doing so. Yet circumcision was never connected to salvation—either by Moses or by Abraham.[64] The Pharisees were promoting a form of spiritual bigotry in Antioch which Peter openly denounced in Jerusalem, largely due to the insight that he gleaned from his strange animal vision and experience with Cornelius.

Abbreviated Gentile Commands?

After hearing testimony from Paul and Barnabas regarding the mass conversion of Gentiles,[65] James felt compelled to quote a portion of Moses' Torah on the heels of Peter's circumcision-salvation speech quoted above, interjecting some interesting opinions of his own. Candidly revealing his position in the matter as personal judgment, James' argument seems to include remarks pertaining to dietary law as well.

> It is my judgment, therefore, that we should not make it difficult for the Gentiles who are turning to God. Instead we should write to them, telling them to abstain from food polluted by idols, from sexual immorality, from the meat of strangled animals and from blood. For Moses has been preached in every city from the earliest times and is read in the synagogues on every Sabbath. (Acts 15:19–21)

This reasoning and judgment of James was apparently unanimously popular in the Jerusalem assembly. Sending a hand-carried letter via

---

64 Genesis 17:10–27; Exodus 12:44, 48; Leviticus 12:3
65 Probably referring to Antioch, Acts 11:20–22.

Paul and Barnabas to the believers of Antioch, Syria, and Cilicia, the 'council' of Jerusalem wrote,

> To the Gentile believers in Antioch, Syria and Cilicia: Greetings.
>
> We have heard that some went out from us without our authorization and disturbed you, troubling your minds by what they said. So we all agreed to choose some men and send them to you with our dear friends Barnabas and Paul—men who have risked their lives for the name of our Lord Jesus Christ. Therefore we are sending Judas and Silas to confirm by word of mouth what we are writing. It seemed good to the Holy Spirit and to us not to burden you with anything beyond the following requirements: You are to abstain from food sacrificed to idols, from blood, from the meat of strangled animals and from sexual immorality. You will do well to avoid these things. (Acts 15:23–29)

Sadly, like Peter's "kill and eat" vision account, such isolated excerpts from Acts have been interpreted to justify a wide variety of lawless behavior over the centuries. Yet the small list described above can hardly be interpreted as a comprehensive listing of do's and don'ts for Gentiles, whether the audience members are new or mature believers. As in the case of Peter's vision, inspection of a few other New Testament texts reveals a much greater context.

Peter's Vision – A Prophecy of Peter

In reading the Jerusalem council account and letter from Acts isolated unto themselves, it is possible to deduce that James and Peter had been a united and inspired duo—leading the way in corrective teaching as the Jerusalem council reached its decision. The great irony of the story, however, is that James and Peter were collectively responsible for leading Antioch's Gentile believers astray some time before their meeting! Though the author of Acts refrains from elaborating on these details, other New Testament texts reveal that Peter had previously sided with overzealous circumcision advocates, who James had initially commissioned to teach in Antioch. These facts surface in Paul's corresponding account written to the Galatians, which again denounced unacceptable Jewish traditions, but did not undermine God's commands given through Moses. Implicating James along with Peter, Paul wrote,

> When Peter came to Antioch, I opposed him to his face, because he was clearly in the wrong. Before certain men came from James, he used to eat with the Gentiles. But when they arrived, he began to draw back and separate himself from the Gentiles because he was afraid of those who belonged to the circumcision group. The other Jews joined him in his hypocrisy, so that by their hypocrisy even Barnabas was led astray.

> When I saw that they were not acting in line with the truth of the gospel, I said to Peter in front of them all, "You are a Jew, yet you live like a Gentile and not like a Jew. How is it, then, that you force Gentiles to follow Jewish customs?" (Gal. 2:11–14)

In light of this Galatians text, the purpose of Peter's rise-kill-eat vision becomes all the more obvious. After all, Paul's writings clearly showed a Peter who was radically different than the one taking the lead at the Jerusalem council meeting – one who was younger, fickle, phobic, and prejudiced. Likewise, Paul revealed how members of Antioch's religious community lacked the ability to distinguish between Moses' law and man-made customs, and overlooked the great importance of being hospitable to new Gentile believers. As such, it would appear from the Galatians text that Peter was enlightened with his vision not for the sake of his lunch menu, but rather for the sake of personal and public correction in arenas of hospitality.

As for Peter's personal character correction, it would appear that Peter's earlier vision in Joppa was insufficient, hence the need for Paul's later rebuke in Antioch.[66] As recorded in Galatians, Peter had a propensity to yield to peer pressure; his national loyalty inspired him to revert to Jewish religious traditions, which included behavior beyond what Moses' law had instructed. Clearly, the meaning of the Acts vision is obscured without considering Peter's character flaws and participation in inappropriate religious bigotry. Therefore, in the same way it is essential to know what Moses and Jesus really said about unclean animals and common foods, it is also crucial to understand Peter's character and experience before the vision, lest the vision be put into improper context. The voice in the vision commanded, "Get up, Peter. Kill and eat!" Yet given Peter's revelation in light of the big picture—including the account of Cornelius and Antioch per the Galatians text, it would be better interpreted as, "Get up, Peter. Make a distinction, and eat with the God-fearing Gentiles who do what is right!" After all, that is exactly how Peter interpreted his vision at the end of the story, and that is exactly how he responded to the revelation.

Four Commandments or Four Men?

By overlooking the greater contexts surrounding the circumcision teachings and Peter's vision, people might be inclined to take the Antioch letter of Acts 15 as a foundation for reducing the duty of believers to four simple, potentially vague, and seemingly arbitrary commandments. Some interpret the Antioch letter as universal and infallible Holy Writ, created to help establish streamlined New Testament doctrines for Gentile churches. But is it correct to infer that the four lone commandments were

---

66 See Galatians 2:1–9 and Acts 11 for a timeline of the Antioch/Jerusalem visit and for Paul/Barnabas connections, plus Galatians 2:10 and Acts 11:29 for a correlating account of a famine relief appeal.

indeed to be regarded as universal and comprehensive—that they were simplified moral mandates for all Gentile believers to live by, starting at that moment and continuing forever? A closer examination of the content and context of the letter demonstrates that this is not a correct interpretation or application of the texts.

At the time the Jerusalem council letter was drafted, the circumstances in Jerusalem and Antioch were complicated and volatile. Jerusalem had been enduring periods of religious persecution, while the Antioch congregation dealt with its own unique set of problems. The assembly in Antioch would be challenged by an influx of persecuted immigrants, the absorption of gentiles, and a variety of new and differing doctrines brought by a medley of teachers. Given such influences and the absence of stability, there would be no telling the amount of damage that the foreign teachers might cause. Consequentially,

Antioch's problems could not be resolved by a single letter decreeing arbitrary observance of four commandments. Given this reality, the letter to Antioch was not written with the intent of delineating four limited commandments applicable to the Gentiles, but rather to introduce four men who would travel to Antioch in the flesh and resolve the confusion among the Gentiles there, representing the consensus reached by the Jerusalem council. The problem was confusion in Antioch; the solution was a four-man team—two hailing from Jerusalem, and two who were well known in Antioch. This cause-effect/problem-solution relationship is outlined in the text below.

> We have heard that some went out from us without our authorization and disturbed you, troubling your minds by what they said. So we all agreed to choose some men and send them to you with our dear friends Barnabas and Paul—men who have risked their lives for the name of our Lord Jesus Christ. Therefore we are sending Judas and Silas to confirm by word of mouth what we are writing. (Acts 15:24–27)

It could be inferred from the opening statement in this passage that the council's greatest concern was to restore tranquility to the congregation of Antioch that Paul and Barnabas reported the conflict to the council. Thus the council's decision to send four men was intended to restore sanity to Antioch and to comfort the people. Two of the four men, Paul and Barnabas, were relatively unaffiliated with the affairs of the Jerusalem council, but were present in Antioch as the circumcision-salvation dispute emerged. As a result, they would be quite cognizant of the parties involved and the doctrinal issues at hand. The remaining two men, Judas (a.k.a. Barsabas, not Judas Iscariot) and Silas, were sent to bear witness to the council's position, thereby representing Jerusalem and confirming the legitimacy of the teaching of Paul and Barnabas, who had already spent a considerable amount of time in Antioch.[67] Furthermore, it stands to reason that Antioch was familiar with Judas and Silas, given their roles as witnesses or emissaries, as described in the letter.

Because of the dispatch of the team of gurus, the council's letter included a very limited set of instructions, and it is obvious that they made no effort to detail and clarify topics preceding its meeting. As such, the letter made no mention of circumcision, no reference to acceptable and unacceptable animal types, and no suggestions on racial or religious segregation in dining environments. It only vaguely mentioned the circumcision-salvation fanatics, who may still have been at large, causing further confusion in the assembly. The letter even failed to mention anything about being 'saved by grace;' it made no comment on the topic of messianic salvation either. To the contrary, these issues – and perhaps many more – were to be resolved by four men after the letter was delivered and the situation assessed.

Letter of Inspiration?

As for the remainder of the Acts letter, it is problematic at best to equate it with universal and infallible Holy Writ created to articulate

---

67 Acts 11:26, 14:21

lasting New Testament doctrines for a Gentile church. As such, the council's letter concludes circumstantially,

> It seemed good to the Holy Spirit and to us not to burden you with anything beyond the following requirements: You are to abstain from food sacrificed to idols, from blood, from the meat of strangled animals and from sexual immorality. You will do well to avoid these things. (Acts 15:28–29)

Lest it be forgotten, the letter was a reaction, created by request and out of necessity in particular circumstances, after major obfuscation of information and corruption of doctrine; it was also addressed specifically to "Gentile believers in Antioch, Syria, and Cilicia." It was delivered along with four expert teachers.[68] To suggest that it applies in its limited capacity to all Gentile churches forevermore is a little like picking up mail sent to someone else and dated 'urgent' or 'time-sensitive' and thinking that the message applies to the third-party interceptor and is complete and eternal. It would be like assuming that a weekly church bulletin or sermon outline is a complete representation of everything uttered from behind the pulpit. It could be compared to fixating upon an answer while completely ignoring the substance of the corresponding question. Obviously, the New Testament audience is left without details as to Antioch's circumstances, needs, inclinations, or demographics, making it that much more difficult to understand any other points of confusion within the Antioch assembly.

Nevertheless, the single concluding 'Holy Spirit' reference might compel many to elevate the authors' authority and infer that the four subsequent instructions were offered as a new and fully comprehensive replacement set of commandments. Yet given its content and construction, equating the letter to communal and Holy Spirit-inspired writ may be problematic. Unlike testimonies from Old Testament prophets, which were always given to or through individuals in the singular and without evidence of democracy or

68 Acts 15:22 identifies Judas and Silas as leaders in Jerusalem.

popular human opinion, the council seems to speak subjectively and more from the perspective of consensus opinion rather than from divine revelation.

The Jerusalem council, a body whose members are unidentified and unknown and therefore unaccountable, clearly and repeatedly employed a 'signature of man' throughout the letter.[69] Like the self-confessed judgment of James preceding it, the nouns and pronouns that the council employed are suggestive. The text contains many phrases emphasizing human origin, involvement, perception, and authority. Phrases demonstrating human initiatives include "we have heard," "out from us," "without our authorization," "we all agreed," "men who have," "therefore we are sending," "word of mouth," "we are writing," and "to us." Surely, the use of blended authority—"it seemed good to the Holy Spirit and to us"—is perhaps the most curious language in the letter, as if it were of critical importance to have God's opinion backed by the council's consent. If that were the case, this would be the first time in Bible history that Almighty God accepted his authority as being equal to that of an anonymous human counsel – or that God would need his authority backed by a human assembly. Surely, remaining anonymous in such a critical affair might be likened to sending the Declaration of Independence without adding signatures. Without witnesses, such a letter would be unlikely to inspire its recipients.

James' Half-Torah

The impact of James' remarks on the council's decision and the letter's content must also be given due consideration. For James made no comments on the subject at hand, namely the circumcision-salvation topic; instead, the teaching of four commandments to the Gentiles was James's suggestion. But why? Where did James and the council get the idea for the four new commandments? Was this revealed to them by the Holy Spirit?

---

69 Acts 15:24–29

At first glance, it might appear as if James were trying to change the subject from circumcision to something else. After all, it is possible that James took individual initiative in dispatching some of Jerusalem's Christian Pharisees without council consent – like he seems to have done earlier while Peter was in Antioch.[70] But in revealing James' advice more carefully, James' suggestion appears to demonstrate a great deal of prudence and insight.

For those familiar with the Torah of Moses, the four commandments given to the Gentiles of Antioch on the recommendation of James will not be viewed as new. All of them, including the injunctions to abstain from idols, blood, meat of strangled animals, and sexual immorality, can be found in the center of Moses' Torah in the book of Leviticus. More specifically, the four commandments can be inferred from a single and central chapter found exactly halfway through the Torah of Moses— Leviticus chapter 19—which includes a summary of prior commandments. These commandments and those surrounding them were not arbitrarily selected; they were foundational to the faith. In fact, these four principles can be easily inferred from even earlier portions of the Bible—all the way back in Genesis.

Following his advice to refer the Gentiles to the very center of Moses' Torah, James makes another curious statement. Not wanting to make things too hard for the new believers of Antioch, James offers some interesting and pertinent reasoning behind his four-commandment recommendation, saying,

> For Moses has been preached in every city from the earliest times and is read in the synagogues on every Sabbath. (Acts 15:21)

James' comment implies firstly that the teachings of Moses would already be familiar to new believers, secondly that they were to continue learning, and finally that synagogues remained legitimate places for doing so! After all, copies of the Scriptures in ancient days were especially scarce

---

70   Galatians 2:12, Acts 15:5

and precious. It's not like the Gideons were stashing mass produced copies of the Hebrew Bible or Greek Septuagint in each hotel room. The William Tyndale and King James Versions were a long way off, as the English language was nonexistent two thousand years ago. Even Guttenberg's printing press was many centuries away from being rolled out. Hand written on sheepskin, the ancient scrolls were expensive to buy and labor intensive to reproduce. Because the scrolls were luxury items, the synagogue was likely to have a set of the divine Hebrew Scriptures handy and available for community use—probably the only copy in town.

From the Acts context, it seems likely that the ex-pagan Gentiles of Antioch, Syria, and Cilicia had little or no foundation in the Scriptures; they didn't even know where to begin! Yet in the local synagogue, not only would they find copies of the texts, but they would be exposed to regular weekly readings of the books of Moses.[71] The synagogue visitation would not only help members of the Gentile community to understand the Bible, which was carefully recorded on Hebrew scrolls, but it would assure that they received the Word in regular and digestible doses through weekly reading cycles, in accordance with ancient traditions. The Gentiles were to learn along with those familiar with the ancient Scripture. Moreover, public synagogue readings would serve both the literate and illiterate. Newcomers could engage in study without feeling left behind forever, since the Jewish tradition of reading the entire works of Moses repeated annually.

Beyond basic study, there were numerous benefits to be realized as a result of Gentile integration into Jewish synagogues. Integration was an essential element in reconciliation and demolishing social barriers between Jews and Gentiles. As the Gentiles integrated themselves among Jews in the synagogues, the divisions and hostility between the believers could begin to dissolve. If an uncircumcised Gentile believer were permitted into a synagogue to learn and worship in accordance with the Hebrew faith, the separation in the dining halls— and throughout the culture—would diminish as well as the Gentiles returned to the covenant and to the God of Abraham, Isaac, and Jacob.

---

71 Acts 15:21

Misunderstandings and long-standing hostilities could be replaced with respect and friendship.

Although it stands to reason that Paul, Barnabas, Silas, and Judas might relay such synagogue attendance recommendations to the Gentile believers, the reverse may also have been true. Paul was well received in some synagogues, while being harshly persecuted in others. He was stoned and left for dead by men from Pisidian Antioch. For this reason, Gentile integration into Jewish synagogues may not have been included as a mandate or even as a recommendation in the Antioch letter. Nevertheless, returning to 'The Heart of the Torah' was exactly what the Jerusalem council was prescribing for the new believers as they reiterated the four commandments in the letter to Antioch. It was the central doctrine of every God-fearing synagogue that revered the law of Moses.

From Sinai's Ten to Antioch's Four to Corinth's Ten

From the standpoint of Christian theology, Paul's rebuke to the believers in Corinth is further evidence that the short four-commandment list sent to Antioch was not complete, universal, or all-encompassing doctrine. Going beyond the Jerusalem council's list of prohibitions, Paul defined wickedness to the Corinthian Gentiles using ten unique terms.

> Do you not know that the wicked will not inherit the kingdom of God? Do not be deceived: Neither the sexually immoral nor idolaters nor adulterers nor male prostitutes nor homosexual offenders nor thieves nor the greedy nor drunkards nor slanderers nor swindlers will inherit the kingdom of God. (1 Cor. 6:9–10)

In contrast with the Jerusalem-Antioch letter list, Paul makes no mention of blood or strangulation to the Corinthians. He does, however, seem to disqualify thieves, drunkards, slanderers, swindlers, and the greedy from the kingdom of heaven. Yet somehow murderers, the covetous, and those disobedient to parents are omitted here. Clearly, neither the Antioch nor the Corinthian letters can be viewed as comprehensive in their scope or complete in their authority. They fail even to cover the breadth of what is described in the Ten Commandments. Surely, such New Testament teachings must be regarded as reiterative and complementary to earlier commandments; they cannot be mistaken for unique revelation introduced to comprehensively replace preexisting moral mandates.

Concluding Peter's Acts with Gentiles

In conclusion, the Acts account surrounding Peter's vision should not be summarized thematically by the one-line "get up Peter; kill and eat" mandate. The story did not begin or end at Peter's vision. It was not about food; it was given to offer specific community integration lessons for Jews and Gentiles alike.

In Joppa, Peter saw a large collection of animals in a vision. He heard a voice that said, "Get up, kill, and eat." He refused and testified that he never ate unclean or defiled animals. Thereafter, Peter was rebuked for making all things unholy, as he rejected them as "common." But he did not understand what the vision meant, and he did not "get up, kill, and eat" or change his diet post-trance.

A righteous Gentile named Cornelius experienced a vision that was concurrent and complementary with Peter's vision. Peter met Cornelius, along with other righteous Gentiles. Cornelius shared his dream with Peter. This first enabled Peter to interpret his own dream and convicted him to confess and repent of his bigotry. While he was forced to eat crow, figuratively speaking, he was not compelled to eat ostriches, pigs, camels, rabbits, frogs, turtles, roaches, or crustaceans, literally speaking. Even Peter's Jerusalem audience who heard his testimony responded to it in like manner.

Paul and Barnabas spent a year teaching in Antioch and made multiple trips to teach there.[72] At some point, Peter met with Paul and Barnabas in Antioch, and he was cordial to righteous Gentile believers.

---

72 Acts 11:26

Over time, James sent Christian Pharisees, who promoted illegitimate circumcision teachings,[73] from Jerusalem to Antioch. As familiar and fellow Jews, Peter befriended them, but he became a little too friendly with them. Unduly influenced by them, Peter stopped eating with "unclean" Gentiles, influencing Barnabas to withdraw. Paul, however, rebuked Peter for his behavior.

Later, after the circumcision-salvation confusion was reintroduced to Antioch, men including Peter, James, Paul, and Barnabas testified before the Jerusalem council. Having learned his lesson from his vision and Paul's rebuke, Peter testified on behalf of the Gentiles, who he no longer belittled and branded as "common." Likewise, James suggested that the Gentiles begin at the center of Moses' Torah to help clarify their misunderstandings. He suggested the opposite of alienating the Gentiles—implying that they should turn to synagogues to learn from Moses' law. The council dispatched Paul, Barnabas, Silas, and Judas for purposes of representation and tasked them to resolve circumcision-salvation doctrine conflicts so that the uncircumcised Gentiles of Antioch would no longer be confused or unjustly alienated.

What should Peter "kill and eat," and with whom should he eat? Discernment would be a central ingredient in Peter's meals in days to follow. He wouldn't drink blood or eat animals killed by strangulation. Maintaining his convictions about animal types, Peter would continue fishing for marine life endowed with fins and scales and keep eating cud-chewing herbivores with split hooves. Yet his perceptions of things unclean would be forever changed, so his policies with respect to human relationships would never be the same. Not only was Peter given the liberty to eat with unwashed hands after fishing or visiting the market— he was also given the freedom to expand his social circles. His dinner company would now include righteous Gentiles.

Just as Jesus never made all foods clean, neither did Peter make them clean through his vision. Peter's lessons, confessions, and instructions were greater than his vision. Rather than "get up, kill, and eat," he would make it a habit to look, listen, and discern. Only then would Peter be happy to sit down, live, and eat!

73 Harvey Falk, *Jesus the Pharisee* (Eugene: Wipf & Stock Publishers, 2003)

Chapter 2 Notes

Chapter 2 Notes

3

The Defiled Food of Paul and Daniel

Eat anything sold in the meat market without raising
questions of conscience, for, 'The earth is the Lord's, and
everything in it.' If some unbeliever invites you to a meal
and you want to go, eat whatever is put before you without
raising questions of conscience.

—1 Cor. 10:25–27

As one who is in the Lord Jesus, I am fully convinced
that no food is unclean in itself. But if anyone regards
something as unclean, then for him it is unclean ... All
food is clean, but it is wrong for a man to eat anything that
causes someone else to stumble.

—Rom. 14:14, 20

esus' hand washing debate and Peter's kill-and-eat vision aren't the only New Testament incidents that are either misunderstood or carelessly handled in order to advocate unkosher worldviews. The gap between cleanliness and godliness is also widened by improper interpretation of Paul's letters to the Corinthians and Romans.[74]

Although the Corinthian and Roman epistles cover different subject matter than do the Mark and Acts accounts, the same illegitimate approach to Bible interpretation is generally used to derive an unclean message from the epistle texts; that is, small excerpts are extracted from the texts, like those cited on the previous page, and interpreted by themselves without due consideration of the surrounding context or earlier Scriptures. In the same way that permission to dine on unclean things is erroneously inferred from Mark and Acts accounts, which were intended to address topics of extra-biblical washing and misappropriated bigotry, the same faulty dining conclusions are indiscriminately drawn from Corinthians and Romans texts, which were written to deal with topics such as idolatry and judgment.

Nevertheless, these dining-related cases extracted from the four different New Testament sources do have something in common—apart from being erroneously interpreted with dispensational biases. Each of these texts, in dealing with eating and food defilement, also deal with a universal theme: dinner company. Thus, to understand New Testament dining doctrines in their entirety, instructions pertaining to mealtime companionship must be considered.

Eating with Sinners or Sinning with Eaters

However discriminating or extreme it may sound from the standpoint of modern Western etiquette and religious norms, Peter wasn't sure where he was supposed to draw the line between himself and

---

74 1 Corinthians 8, 10:23–31; Romans 14

the righteous Gentiles of Antioch. According to the Acts and Galatians accounts, Peter was vacillating between an endearing friendship and a distant and informal religious affiliation. Per Paul's rebuke and his own subsequent animal vision, Peter learned that he had alienated the Antioch Gentile believers without just cause. However, the Jerusalem council's advice to Antioch, to abstain from "food polluted by idols,"[75] should also be considered in context and factored into interpretation of the texts. Had the Antioch Gentiles been engaged in paganism, worshiping and feasting to idols, Peter and his non-idol-worshiping Pharisaic counterparts would have valid reasons to withdraw themselves from them. Confronted with a populous that had been steeped in idolatry, how was a righteous Jew like Peter to respond? Should he be expected to eat with Gentiles in Antioch if they were eating foods offered to idols?

With Paul's dilemmas being very similar to those encountered by Peter in Antioch, Paul's letters to the Corinthian and Roman communities specifically addressed issues of eating and companionship within idolatrous cultures. Hosting two prominent harbors, transient sailors, and the temple of Aphrodite (the Greek goddess of love), the city of Corinth was also regarded to be among the most morally degenerate of the Roman Empire, notorious for its pagan festivals and temple prostitutes. Logically, one of the challenges that Paul faced was teaching new Roman believers how to divorce themselves from pagan practices and influences without completely isolating and alienating themselves from rest of society—which would include other new believers.

Of course, the question of who to associate with is no trivial matter, especially given the possible implications of gathering members of mixed political, religious, and ethnic factions. Dining environments with such diversity can be pregnant with tension; it is inevitable that mustering people of drastically different cultural, moral, and hygienic standards will result in some measure of conflict. Consequently, the line between *sinning with eaters* and *eating with sinners* might be difficult to perceive.

---

75 Acts 15:20

Kosher Dining Hall Company

Of course, first-century dining-company problems were not unique to pagan places like Antioch or Corinth; similar problems were prominent in regions of Judea and Samaria, where pagan idolatry was scarce and where a number of Jewish factions shaped the religious landscape. Yet even within Israel's borders, Jesus had been discredited by religious authorities because he showed hospitality to the "sinners," the dregs of society.

Although the gospel of Luke does not appear to differentiate between a degenerate Jew and a degenerate Gentile, Jesus' remarks to the religious authorities provide guidance on how to qualify an outcast or "sinner" as someone righteous enough to accept as a dinner guest. After being criticized for his choice of company, Jesus responded with a parable to defend his companions and his relationship with them.

> Now the tax collectors and "sinners" were all gathering around to hear him. But the Pharisees and the teachers of the law muttered, "This man welcomes sinners and eats with them." Then Jesus told them this parable: "Suppose one of you has a hundred sheep and loses one of them. Does he not leave the ninety-nine in the open country and go after the lost sheep until he finds it? And when he finds it, he joyfully puts it on his shoulders and goes home. Then he calls his friends and neighbors together and says, 'Rejoice with me; I have found my lost sheep.' I tell you that in the same way there will be more rejoicing in heaven over one sinner who repents than over ninety-nine righteous persons who do not need to repent." (Luke 15:1–7)

Although the content of Jesus' dining conversation with his disreputable company cannot be deduced from the short gospel text, his concluding comments suggest that his companions sought him out for his teaching, that his teaching was corrective, and that encouraging repentance was the motive for his relationship with "sinners." Therefore, anyone open to corrective teaching and willing to repent might be categorized as worthwhile company. Conversely, those blinded by pride and convinced that they had it all together might better be categorized as lost in self-righteousness.

Approved Behavioral Bigotry

Likewise, in his letter to the Corinthians, Paul offers a simple listing of qualifications for dining companions, sternly warning his audience about associating with the self-righteous, as Jesus did.[76] Above all, Paul instructed his audience to shun hypocrites who masquerade as fellow believers, especially during mealtime.

> "But now I am writing you that you must not associate with anyone who calls himself a brother but is sexually immoral or greedy, an idolater or a slanderer, a drunkard or a swindler. With such a man do not even eat." (1 Cor. 5:11)

In contrast to the illegitimate circumcision-based schism that Peter and the Pharisees created in Antioch, Paul did not promote dining division over circumcision or national heritage. Instead, Paul insisted that believers avoid dining with self-righteous hypocrites, including the idolatrous in his listing of unwelcome company. For all practical purposes, Paul's advice to the Corinthian believers was consistent with the Jerusalem council's instruction to the Gentiles of Antioch to "abstain from 'meats' offered to idols."[77] After his "kill and eat" vision, there is no reason to believe that Peter would have dining standards differing from Paul's; Peter would not see a religious duty to accept *all* persons, including idolaters and hypocrites, but rather to accept all persons who did what was right. As Peter learned through unusual circumstances, social expectations were to apply as equally to longstanding Jewish believers as they were to new Gentile believers.

---

76 Luke 18:9
77 Acts 15:29, KJV

Corinth's Idolatrous History

Paul's reference to idolatry in chapter 5 of his first letter to the Corinthians was not an isolated allusion to Corinthian idolatry. In fact, Paul opened his letter by accusing the congregation of idolizing those who were teaching them—be it himself, Peter, Apollos, or even Christ.[78] Moreover, Paul reminded the Corinthian believers of their idolatrous reputation, saying,

> "You know that when you were pagans, somehow or other you were influenced and led astray to mute idols." (1 Cor. 12:2)

Paul's Corinthian admonition, which was cited in the prior chapter to debunk morally problematic "four lone Gentile commandments of Acts" dogma, is also indicative that the congregation was vulnerable to idolatry. As such, idolatry was listed among the deadliest of sins.

> "Do you not know that the wicked will not inherit the kingdom of God? Do not be deceived: Neither the sexually immoral nor idolaters nor adulterers nor male prostitutes nor homosexual offenders nor thieves nor the greedy nor drunkards nor slanderers nor swindlers will inherit the kingdom of God." (1 Cor. 6:9–10)

The Corinthian congregation, however, had apparently repented of its idolatry. Recalling the Corinthians' idolatrous behavior as something in the past tense, Paul reminds them in the next verse,

> "And that is what some of you were." (1 Cor. 6:11)

Thus, when Paul began to write about food and idol feasts in his first letter to the Corinthians, he was hardly speaking hypothetically or introducing a topic at random. To the contrary, Paul was addressing

---

78 1 Corinthians 1:12

a real congregation of immature believers. Among the congregation, there were recovering idolaters who remained immersed in a pagan religious culture—day in and day out. In fact, the Corinthians were so immature and tainted by the culture that they openly tolerated incest within the congregation.[79] So, however bizarre the idea of idol feasts might seem to the Western mind, it is important to remember that idolatrous dining celebrations were every bit as real in Corinth as they were when the Israelites worshiped the golden calf at the base of Mount Sinai.

The Corinthian Departure from Idolatry

However, Paul's Corinthian audience had embarked on a path of repentance; they were departing from pantheistic and pagan idolatry as they were embracing the truth of monotheism. Yet however repentant the Corinthians may have been or hoped to become, their minds would undoubtedly be ingrained with many pagan ideas, and it is highly improbable that they would shed all of their idolatrous reasoning and customs overnight. They needed time to unlearn their pagan doctrines as they learned new scriptural truths from scratch. Given their newfound and limited knowledge, Paul needed to assure the Corinthians that any ceremonial pomp associated with idolatrous feasts and foods was not only meaningless, but without physical or spiritual consequence— provided that they were not participating in such pagan ceremonies themselves. Therefore, Paul explained to the more mature members of the Corinthian congregation,

> Now about food sacrificed to idols: We know that we all possess knowledge. Knowledge puffs up, but love builds up. The man who thinks he knows something does not yet know as he ought to know. But the man who loves God is known by God.

---

79 i.e., son/mother or son/stepmother sexual relations, 1 Corinthians 5:2

So then, about eating food sacrificed to idols: We know that an idol is nothing at all in the world and that there is no God but one. For even if there are so-called gods, whether in heaven or on earth (as indeed there are many "gods" and many "lords"), yet for us there is but one God, the Father, from whom all things came and for whom we live. (1 Cor. 8:1–6)

With his words above, Paul clearly rejects the idols' ability to corrupt food, but he obviously did not expect all Corinthian believers to instantly arrive at the same conclusion. Instead, he expected it would take time for some of them to shed their superstitions, which had been engrained into their minds over the course of decades by means of subtle traditions and everyday rituals. They needed time to unlearn many things they had mistaken for truth. After figuratively believing for decades that the world was flat, so to speak, they would not all grasp the principles and implications of global geography and spherical geometry in a single day. So, in dealing with indoctrinated believers who had little knowledge or discernment, Paul was particularly sensitive and encouraged patience.

Weak Consciences

For the sake of ignorant and undiscerning Corinthians, Paul continued by reminding the more knowledgeable members of his audience of the impotence of idols, as well as the gullibility of some members in their congregation.

But not everyone knows this. Some people are still so accustomed to idols that when they eat such food they think of it as having been sacrificed to an idol, and since their conscience is weak, it is defiled. But food does not bring us near to God;[80] we are no worse if we do not eat, and no better if we do.

Be careful, however, that the exercise of your freedom does not become a stumbling block to the weak. For if anyone with a weak conscience sees you who have this knowledge eating in an idol's temple,[81] won't he be emboldened to eat what has been sacrificed to idols? (1 Cor. 8:7–10)

Once again, Paul was not making appeals on behalf of the indifferent; the people of weak conscience[82] to whom he referred were those with poor discernment or limited powers of perception. He did not want those capable of discerning and avoiding idolatry to set a bad example for those who were ignorant or couldn't tell the difference between right and wrong. Even though it is not possible to defile food with an idol, Paul didn't want an immature person with a so-called "weak conscience" to be led back into paganism as a result of blasé behavior by those who understood this truth. Paul was instructing the more knowledgeable believers to be sensitive to the superstitious and ignorant, lest they revert to practicing their pagan customs.

---

80 The term קרבן (*qorban*, Strong's H7133) means something "brought near the altar" or to God; it is used to describe Hebrew sacrifices and fellowship offerings in Leviticus and Numbers. Because Paul suggests that the *food* involved with sacrifices contained no spiritual or mystical properties, it stands to reason that it was instead the sacrificial act that made the closeness with God possible. A reciprocal relationship was likely inferred by pagan cultures whereby the food was thought to be the path to communion or fellowship with the deity. Thus the former pagans would find it difficult to make such subtle distinctions as new believers.

81 Like government buildings erected today, so too were many public buildings of the Roman period adorned with idolatrous imagery; thus they would logically be perceived as "idol temples" by Corinthian and Roman believers. By today's standards, the scenario described might be comparable to eating a "brown bag" lunch in a courthouse or capitol building, which often incorporate pagan themes and imagery.

82 Strong's G4893, συνείδησις (suneidēsis), derived from Strong's G4894, συνείδω (suneidō), which is translated as *conscience,* also implies perception or moral decisiveness, understanding, discernment, or awareness.

Sacred Cows versus Golden Calves

As Paul explained to the Corinthians, there is a profound difference between eating foods offered to idols and offering foods to idols; the real distinction lies in who is doing the offering and worshiping. Idolatry, after all, is in the heart and mind of the beholder. Given this principle, a starving man in India is by no means obligated to refrain from eating what his fellow countrymen believe to be a sacred cow. Misdirected worship won't pollute the beef of the impoverished, unless the impoverished participates in misdirected worship. In other words, sacred cows can make great steaks.

In a similar manner, Paul said it was acceptable to eat a cow that someone else held to be sacred—as long as doing so didn't cause a fellow believer grief and as long as it wasn't construed as a feast in honor of an idol. The congregation of Corinth, much like the congregation of Antioch, was warned against making idolatrous offerings and socially joining themselves to those who did so. However, Paul did not warn against a believer eating or touching foods that someone else had offered to idols, although some ignorant believers incorrectly assumed that such foods were defiled by idolatry.

Polluting Food, People, and Translations

Despite Paul's clear Corinthian teaching on the distinctions, some still interpret certain New Testament texts with superstitious notions, believing that food *can* be defiled by idolatry. For example, certain texts in Acts from the New International Version would lead readers to believe that there are indeed sacred cows and that it is indeed possible to pollute food by idols. The erroneous claim that foods are polluted through association with idols appears in the translation of the verse where James offers his opinion to the council in Jerusalem.

> Instead we should write to them, telling them to abstain
> from food polluted by idols, from sexual immorality, from

the meat of strangled animals and from blood. (Acts 15:20 NIV)

Nevertheless, Paul's teaching to the Corinthians does not support the notion that foods can be polluted by idols, nor do other translations of Acts, which better convey the message of the ancient Greek. For example, the same Acts verse in the King James translation excludes mention of food, reading more closely relative to the original Greek.

But that we write unto them, that they abstain from pollutions of idols, and from fornication, and from things strangled, and from blood. (Acts 15:20 KJV)

James' suggestion, as quoted in verse 20, included the Greek terms αλισγεμα (al-is'-ghem-ah),[83] meaning "defilement" or "pollution," and ειδωλον (i'-do-lon),[84] meaning "image," "idol," or "heathen god," but there is no reference to *food* in the Greek! In this verse, James warns the people to avoid becoming defiled by heathen gods. However, it is of critical importance to note that the Greek text does not mention making offerings to them, nor does James refer to food—or to food becoming corrupt from such offering.

Acts of Idolatrous Worship

While James' advice to avoid being defiled by foreign gods was profound and remains sound, the Jerusalem council did not reiterate this advice verbatim in their letter. Whereas James was defining *what* to avoid, as articulated in the Acts quote above, the council went on to more pointedly describe *how* new believers might avoid the pollution that James described. In other words, where James was advising that the people avoid *defilement by* idols, the council gave more practical and less

---

83 Strong's G234
84 Strong's G1497

theoretical advice to these believers, telling them with greater specificity to stop *making offerings to* idols.

Unfortunately, compounding the translation obfuscation problems, both the New International Version and the King James text refer to *foods* in conjunction with pagan sacrifices several verses later, although there is no mention of *defilement* or *pollution* made in conjunction with the alleged food reference. Slightly modifying James' initial recommendation, the Jerusalem council's advice to Antioch is conveyed as cited below.

> That ye abstain from meats offered to idols, and from blood, and from things strangled, and from fornication: from which if ye keep yourselves, ye shall do well. Fare ye well. (Acts 15:29 KJV)

Although the translations both mention offering "meats" or "foods"[85] to idols, it is of greater importance to note that the original Greek text makes no clear reference to meat, food, or eating. This can be deduced from the Jerusalem council's reference to ειδωλοθυτον (i-do-loth'-oo-ton)[86] in verse 29, meaning an "idolatrous offering." Although this term *may* convey food offerings, it is significant that the term may be used much more generically, encompassing *anything* offered by means of fire or slaughter.[87] Thus, the original Greek of verse 29 contains no particular reference to eating and so does not support the literal King James translation of ειδωλοθυτον (i-do-loth'-oo-ton) as an idolatrous "meat" offering. Furthermore, as translated, it might be mistakenly interpreted in an eating sense as "abstain from meats," as opposed to a worship sense, as in "abstain from offering to idols," as the Greek more clearly instructs.

---

85 Refer to page 39 for NIV translation citation.

86 Strong's G1494

87 Strong's G1494 is derived from G1497 (idol or heathen god) and G2380 (possibly smoke or something sacrificed by fire or by slaughter).

Acts of Defilement

With a proper understanding of the Greek terms, the subtle distinctions between James' suggestion in verse 20 and the council's official recommendation in verse 29 become useful in discerning a collective meaning. If the people stopped making offerings to idols (regardless of what they offered), they would avoid being corrupted by heathen gods. After all, it is completely reasonable to believe that people might be corrupted by the *worship* of heathen gods—but to advocate the notion that an idol can defile foods or other objects is to fall victim to superstition. This is essentially the same superstition that Paul was trying to dismantle in Corinth,[88] as his letter as cited on page 60 demonstrates, where some people thought that the object of the idol sacrifice was capable of corrupting a person—not realizing that the true danger was in the act of offering.

Not surprisingly, the same 'idolatrous food defilement' dogma inferred by Corinthians and implied by Acts translations is essentially the same as that held by Pharisees in the Mark 7 account; both were formulated by unfamiliarity with the Torah of Moses. After all, the Torah includes specific commandments against idolatry; it also describes a number of ways in which food could be defiled. Food could become defiled by contact with unclean things,[89] contact with unclean persons,[90] or being in close proximity to the dead.[91] In stark contrast, the consequence of idol worship was not food pollution, but destruction and ejection from the land.[92] Also, James' revelations pertaining to corruption from affiliation with heathen gods[93] are in perfect agreement with Moses' warning about evil spirits defiling the soul.[94] Therefore, the spiritual implications of eating foods sacrificed to idols should be considered to be just as moot as eating food with unwashed hands.

---

88 1 Corinthians 8
89 Leviticus 7:19, Leviticus 11:31–38
90 Deuteronomy 26:14
91 Numbers 19:14–15
92 Deuteronomy 4:23–27
93 Acts 15:20
94 Leviticus 19:31

Ancient Israelite Reruns

While the idol itself, along with food dedicated to it, was rendered harmless by Paul and the Torah, Paul repeatedly warned against participating in idol feasts, as did Moses. Dedicating an entire chapter to discouraging idolatry, Paul admonished the Corinthians by recalling ancient Israel's golden calf feast at the foot of Mount Sinai,

> "Do not be idolaters, as some of them were; as it is written: 'The people sat down to eat and drink and got up to indulge in pagan revelry'" (1 Cor. 10:7).

Given this context, Paul reiterated his concerns about breaking bread at an idolatrous celebration, as attendees "communed" with one another—as well as with spirits invoked at such festivals. Discouraging people from participating in or even appearing at such festivals, Paul reasoned with his audience,

> Consider the people of Israel: Do not those who eat the sacrifices participate in the altar? Do I mean then that a sacrifice offered to an idol is anything, or that an idol is anything? No, but the sacrifices of pagans are offered to demons, not to God, and I do not want you to be participants with demons. You cannot drink the cup of the Lord and the cup of demons too; you cannot have a part in both the Lord's table and the table of demons. (1 Cor. 10:18–21)

So, writing succinctly and exclusively about idolatry to a congregation still repenting from paganism, Paul stated:

- ✓ Idols are by nature impotent, harmless, and useless.
- ✓ Food cannot be defiled by proximity to idols.
- ✓ Food cannot be polluted via idolatrous ceremony.
- ✓ Food peripheral to idolatrous activity remains edible.

✓ Food from idol feasts should be avoided if it troubles an immature brother or inclines him to revert to idolatry.

✓ Participation in idol worship or feasts is unacceptable.

✓ Believers practicing idolatry should be excommunicated.

✓ Evil spirits present at idolatrous feasts can defile people.

Morally Benign Venues

In teaching these many things to the Corinthians, Paul never contends against any of Moses' dietary teachings. Regardless, from a single excerpt of Corinthians, many dispensationalists have extrapolated God's line of dining decency to an end point far off Moses' curve, incorrectly claiming that Paul concludes with anti-kosher rhetoric. Forgetting that Paul is making concluding remarks on idolatry, and failing to consider that Paul makes no mention of the animal types that Moses forbade, the Corinthians citation below is nevertheless assumed to justify indiscriminate diets, where everything from the buffet table is regarded as permissible.

> "Everything is permissible"—but not everything is beneficial. "Everything is permissible"—but not everything is constructive. Nobody should seek his own good, but the good of others.

> Eat anything sold in the meat market without raising questions of conscience, for, "The earth is the Lord's, and everything in it." If some unbeliever invites you to a meal and you want to go, eat whatever is put before you without raising questions of conscience.

> But if anyone says to you, "This has been offered in sacrifice," then do not eat it, both for the sake of the man who told you and for conscience' sake—the other man's conscience, I mean, not yours. For why should my freedom be judged

by another's conscience? If I take part in the meal with thankfulness, why am I denounced because of something I thank God for? So whether you eat or drink or whatever you do, do it all for the glory of God. (1 Cor. 10:23–31)

While maintaining continuity in subject matter, Paul's instructions to the Corinthians are perfectly congruent with Peter's words, James' opinion, the Jerusalem council's advice, Jesus' teachings, and the mandates of Moses. Paul does not undermine dietary laws whatsoever, even though he approves the consumption of surplus food obtained from either idol temples or idolatrous feasts. Thus, Paul permitted believers to eat things that were available in a morally neutral marketplace, which should not be equated to morally deplorable pagan feasts. Likewise, Paul encouraged them to feel at home as they accepted the hospitality of unbelievers—though he wasn't giving them a green light to eat with idolaters at pagan festivals. Furthermore, Paul remained sensitive to the new believer's limited perception and discernment of food defilement. He insisted that the food, whatever it might be, and with whomever it might be shared, should be received in thanksgiving to God. Eating with thanksgiving to the one true God guarantees that idol worship is anything but the focal point of the meal.

Distorting Anything and Eating Whatever

Nevertheless, two Corinthians excerpts are commonly used to advocate an unkosher Christian diet. Paul instructed the Corinthians to:

- ✓ Eat anything sold in the meat market without raising questions of conscience, for, 'The earth is the Lord's, and everything in it.'
- ✓ Eat whatever is put before you without raising questions of conscience.

Even if these concluding statements are isolated from their contexts in favor of an unkosher worldview, they still leave the reader with obvious logical problems. After all, if English words like *whatever* and *anything* are taken literally and unconditionally, the meaning of the texts could extend into the absurd, beyond the scope of animal meat, even into the realm of inorganic materials. Of course, nobody would be expected to eat a ceramic dish along with the meal, nor would anyone eat metal or wooden utensils often sold in meat markets. Likewise, Paul was neither advocating the consumption of blood nor consenting to cannibalism. Thus, indiscriminately eating "whatever is served" or "whatever you find in the market" is not consistent with the greater context of Corinthians. If conditions are not imposed on "whatever" or "anything," then eating meat from strangled animals, consuming blood, or even cannibalism would become permissible. Paul isn't telling the Corinthian congregation to start eating anything and everything that moves or sits. He was not recommending the ingestion of unclean animals any more than he was encouraging believers to try eating animal waste, shards of glass, or poison because these things were available in the marketplace or at their dinner table.

Unclean Teachings of Romans

Like his instructions to the Corinthians, Paul's letter to the Romans is also mishandled—being twisted and extracted from its greater context. Advocating unkosher dining and a system of moral relativism, dispensational theologians distill teachings into simplistic food arguments, using three verses from Romans.

> One man's faith allows him to eat everything, but another man, whose faith is weak, eats only vegetables. (Rom 14:2)

> As one who is in the Lord Jesus, I am fully convinced that no food is unclean in itself. But if anyone regards something as unclean, then for him it is unclean. (Rom. 14:14)

Do not destroy the work of God for the sake of food. All food is clean, but it is wrong for a man to eat anything that causes someone else to stumble. (Rom. 14:20)

Given the precedent established by kosher exegesis of numerous Mark, Acts, and Corinthians verses, it is unreasonable to surmise that Paul's teachings to the Romans were ever intended to inspire them to deviate from Mosaic dietary standards. However, in order to arrive at a kosher interpretation of Romans, these verses must also be considered in their greater context.

Judgment, Jews, and Gentiles

The letter to the Romans, written to a mixed congregation of Jews and Gentiles, speaks extensively to the topic of judgment. Paul articulates both divine and human expectations therein. He begins by recalling the historical depravity of mankind, declaring God's wrath to the idolatrous generations.

The wrath of God is being revealed from heaven against all the godlessness and wickedness of men who suppress the truth by their wickedness, since what may be known about God is plain to them, because God has made it plain to them. (Rom. 1:18–19)

Although they claimed to be wise, they became fools and exchanged the glory of the immortal God for images made to look like mortal man and birds and animals and reptiles. (Rom. 1:22–23)

After introducing his letter to the Romans with a brief overview of a depraved and idolatrous faction of humanity, Paul makes a rather abrupt transition, using the preamble to warn and even accuse Roman believers of hypocritical judgment. He even likened some of them to the idolaters and adulterers of antiquity.

> Although they know God's righteous decree that those who do such things deserve death, they not only continue to do these very things but also approve of those who practice them. You, therefore, have no excuse, you who pass judgment on someone else, for at whatever point you judge the other, you are condemning yourself, because you who pass judgment do the same things. (Rom. 1:32, 2:1)

As Paul continued his dissertation to the congregation in Rome, his rebuke was mostly directed toward the Jewish believers there. His rebuke was not incited by what the Jews believed or what they were teaching, as was the case in Antioch or Jerusalem; his words condemned their inconsistent behavior. Praising the Jews' knowledge—but not their behavior—Paul asked rhetorically,

> Now you, if you call yourself a Jew; if you rely on the law and brag about your relationship to God; if you know his will and approve of what is superior because you are instructed by the law; if you are convinced that you are a guide for the blind, a light for those who are in the dark, an instructor of the foolish, a teacher of infants, because you have in the law the embodiment of knowledge and truth— you, then, who teach others, do you not teach yourself? You who preach against stealing, do you steal? You who say that people should not commit adultery, do you commit adultery? You who abhor idols, do you rob temples? You who brag about the law, do you dishonor God by breaking the law? (Rom. 2:17–23)

However awkward or even anti-Semitic Paul's impersonal interrogation of the Jews may seem, he wasn't obsessed with condemning them in his letter to the Romans, nor did he unconditionally condemn them all. Much like the Hebrew prophets, he made his condemnation conditional. Underscoring God's justice, Paul reminded the Roman believers of God's grace, saying that there would be "glory, honor, and peace for everyone who does good"[95] and that those who obeyed the law would be declared righteous in God's sight.[96]

The topic of judgment would remain especially pertinent to the Jewish believers, however, as Paul continued his letter. After all, the Jews within the Roman congregation were familiar with the law of Moses and therefore knew better, whereas the Gentiles were more likely to be oblivious in their behavior, being biblically illiterate from the start, incapable of applying biblical principles to judicial matters. In other words, the Gentiles were forced to rely on conscience, which might have been numbed[97] from neglect or tainted by surrounding customs and peoples, as opposed to the divine and morally absolute Scriptures, with which the Jews were fully acquainted. The majority of Paul's letter to the Romans is written with such basic Jewish and Gentile differences in mind.

Against the backdrop of such Jew/Gentile schisms, the letter to the Romans is wide in scope—covering God's autonomy in judgment, faith and faithful living, the law of Moses and lawful living, as well as man's justification and means to salvation. Yet perhaps most pertinent to justice-related matters, it deals with the reconciliation between the Jews and lost tribes of Israel, otherwise referred to as "wild olive branches."[98] So when Paul writes to the Roman congregation, he logically speaks of this reconciliation between the Jews and other "Gentile" Israelite remnants. This is the greater context of Romans.

---

95 Romans 2:10
96 Romans 2:13
97 1 Timothy 4:2 refers to searing the conscience.
98 Thistles or other fruitless varieties cannot be grafted into olive trees.

Roman Rule and Revenge

Paul's food admonitions, which emerge later in the letter to the Romans, must therefore be considered from greater contexts of judgment and reconciliation. Before making statements about dining expectations, Paul begins by encouraging the Roman congregation in humility and forgiveness.

> For by the grace given me I say to every one of you: Do not think of yourself more highly than you ought, but rather think of yourself with sober judgment, in accordance with the measure of faith God has given you...

> Be devoted to one another in brotherly love. Honor one another above yourselves...

> Live in harmony with one another. Do not be proud, but be willing to associate with people of low position. Do not be conceited. Do not repay anyone evil for evil. Be careful to do what is right in the eyes of everybody. If it is possible, as far as it depends on you, live at peace with everyone. Do not take revenge, my friends, but leave room for God's wrath, for it is written: "'It is mine to avenge; I will repay,' says the Lord." (Rom. 12:3, 10, 16–19)

After discouraging vengeance, it stands to reason that Paul makes an appeal to submit instead to the governing authorities in such matters, be they secular or religious. Divine justice, after all, must be in the hands of governing officials, who have been appointed within communities to render judgments and prescribe punishments; true justice is not appointed to vigilantes emotionally motivated by vengeance.

Roman Rejection

Thus, Paul's appeal to governing authorities is particularly relevant in contexts where law and judgment are being discussed. In other words, Paul reminded the Corinthian believers of the rule of law within a religious and Roman community—just before he introduces his material on eating.

> Everyone must submit himself to the governing authorities, for there is no authority except that which God has established. The authorities that exist have been established by God. (Rom. 13:1)

Also, before discussing foods that are assumed to be defiled, Paul presents a hypothetical case, making an unusual example of a vegetarian believer.

> Accept him whose faith is weak, without passing judgment on disputable matters. One man's faith allows him to eat everything, but another man, whose faith is weak, eats only vegetables. The man who eats everything must not look down on him who does not, and the man who does not eat everything must not condemn the man who does, for God has accepted him. Who are you to judge someone else's servant? To his own master he stands or falls. And he will stand, for the Lord is able to make him stand. (Rom. 14:1–4)

Obviously, Paul's directions in Romans chapter 14 have more to do with mercy and less to do with food. This overarching mercy principle is consistent given Paul's social relations emphasis in chapter 12, and is consistent with Paul's reminder about government responsibilities in chapter 13. Focusing on mercy, Paul does not want the Romans to harshly condemn people for the sake of trivial things.

Roman Vegetarians—Weak in Faith?

Of course, the hypothetical case of veganism described in the opening verses of Romans chapter 14 could be readily correlated with a number of different Scripture passages. First of all, the fact that Moses repeatedly encouraged the consumption of meat as part of the regular diet as well as festive fellowship sacrifices must be considered.[99] Moses' law also commanded that animal meat be part of the priests' diet.[100] And lest it be forgotten, the Passover festival required that a family eat a lamb in its entirety.[101] So, according to Moses' writings, vegans or vegetarians might be described as people whose "faith is weak" if their diets are based on moral convictions—as they would not know, accept, nor observe such principles. Also, Paul may well have been alluding to these particular commandments of Moses when he referred to them as "disputable matters," since there were no consequences outlined in Moses' Torah for anyone who failed to eat meat, whether in a festive assembly or home setting. Furthermore, the "faith is weak" phrase that Paul uses in Romans to describe the vegans seems to correlate with the "weak conscience" description in earlier Corinthian excerpts, implying a lack of understanding.

The account of Daniel offers another example involving a man who restricted his diet to vegetables, as did his three friends, Hananiah, Mishael, and Azariah.[102] Yet these four men, especially Daniel, hardly fit Paul's description of vegans or vegetarians having "weak faith." To the contrary, it was Daniel's strong faith that gave him the conviction not to eat the king's food in the first place—even risking life and limb—lest he be "defiled" by it. Furthermore, Daniel, along with Noah and Job, is described as one of the giants of the faith by the prophet Ezekiel.[103] Therefore, it is not fair to draw parallels between Daniel's dining decisions and Paul's letter to the Romans about a brother of

---

99 Leviticus 3, 7; Leviticus 11; Deuteronomy 12:15
100 Leviticus 8:31
101 Exodus 12
102 Daniel 1:11–12
103 Ezekiel 14:14

"weak faith," especially since Daniel resorted to the vegetarian diet specifically to avoid unclean royal foods.

However, the story of Cain and Abel also seems to encompass a case of vegetarian strife much like the scenario Paul describes in Romans. While Abel brought an animal from the flock, Cain worked the soil and instead brought produce from the earth as an offering. For reasons not identified with perfect clarity, God did not look favorably on Cain's offering, but he accepted Abel's. Although the text does not say that Abel expressed disapproval of Cain's offering of fruits or vegetables,[104] the possibility nevertheless does exist. Did Abel criticize Cain's offering, thereby provoking Cain's contempt, before being murdered? Regardless of Abel's actions, it remains safe to say that Cain was the brother of weaker faith—exhibiting vegetarian preferences—similar to what the Romans text describes.

Defiled and Unclean in the Mind of the Beholder

After alluding to Old Testament dietary precepts, Paul continues in his reasoning to the Romans, focusing on the theme of unwarranted judgment or condemnation, while using the vegetarian with weak faith as an example.

> You, then, why do you judge your brother? Or why do you look down on your brother? For we will all stand before God's judgment seat. (Rom. 14:10)

So it is from the context of illegitimate judgment that Paul mentions unclean food. He continues, maintaining the theme of unwarranted condemnation.

Therefore let us stop passing judgment on one another.

---

104 Although Abel accuses Cain of stealing wool and meat from his flock, according to Jasher 1:19–20.

Instead, make up your mind not to put any stumbling block or obstacle in your brother's way.

As one who is in the Lord Jesus, I am fully convinced that no food is unclean in itself. But if anyone regards something as unclean, then for him it is unclean. If your brother is distressed because of what you eat, you are no longer acting in love. Do not by your eating destroy your brother for whom Christ died...

Do not destroy the work of God for the sake of food. All food is clean, but it is wrong for a man to eat anything that causes someone else to stumble. It is better not to eat meat or drink wine or to do anything else that will cause your brother to fall. (Rom. 14:13–15, 20–21)

Surely, it is unreasonable to assert that Paul's concluding remarks on food in these citations are unrelated to the vegetarian condemnation scenario he had presented earlier. Just as the ex-idolater of Corinth was superstitious about foods exposed to idols or idolatrous ceremonies, so too did the vegetarian self-impose illegitimate perceptions, be they moral or religious, about the prudence of the use of animals for food. Therefore, the Corinthian (idol-based) and Roman (animal-based) perceptions of the defilement of food were almost one and the same; such perceptions of defilement were equally unfounded, originating from someone with a weak conscience, having weak faith, or a lack of discernment—not understanding what the Scriptures said about such foods.

Defiled Foods and Defiled Bodies

In his remarks to the Romans as cited above, Paul wasn't talking about someone who was ignorant of Moses' kosher instructions, rejecting food based on unfounded superstition. As a point of comparison, the prophet Daniel did not declare all foods clean that were presented to him in Babylon; he did not eat what was set before him without raising questions of conscience. To the contrary, Daniel perceived that the royal Babylonian food was unclean or defiled, and he boldly identified it as such.[105] Moses' law provides ample evidence to affirm that Daniel's perceptions were based on kosher reasoning.[106]

First of all, the circumstances of Daniel's protest can be regarded as an ancient science experiment. He and his three friends served as a control group on a restricted diet, whereas the rest of the royal subjects of the experiment would literally eat like kings—that is, uncleanly and irresponsibly! Describing Daniel and his Jewish friends as extremely intelligent and in good physical condition, the account reads,

> Then the king ordered Ashpenaz, chief of his court officials, to bring in some of the Israelites from the royal family and the nobility—young men without any physical defect, handsome, showing aptitude for every kind of learning, well informed, quick to understand, and qualified to serve in the king's palace. He was to teach them the language and literature of the Babylonians. The king assigned them a daily amount of food and wine from the king's table. (Dan. 1:3–5)

Daniel and friends, educated, bright, and healthy, conscientiously objected to consuming the royal diet for fear of defilement. They understood Moses as well as cause-effect relationships. They were capable of discerning what sort of things were being prepared for dinner in Babylonian kitchens, and they knew they wanted nothing to do with them.

Putting his aptitude, political skill, and even scientific knowledge to good use, Daniel requested a temporary exemption from the king's

---

105 Daniel 1:8

106 Unclean food might refer to a food type prohibited by Leviticus 11, whereas defiled food might refer to an acceptable or clean food type that had been contaminated by contact with foods of unclean types, e.g., Leviticus 11:33. Neither was to be eaten.

food; he even went so far as to propose that a controlled experiment be conducted, along with a third-party physical exam, to measure the success of each diet plan.

> 'Please test your servants for ten days: Give us nothing but vegetables to eat and water to drink. Then compare our appearance with that of the young men who eat the royal food, and treat your servants in accordance with what you see.' So he agreed to this and tested them for ten days. At the end of the ten days they looked healthier and better nourished than any of the young men who ate the royal food. (Dan. 1:12–15)

As the text indicates, Daniel's experiment and objection was twofold; not only did he reject the royal unclean food, but he also abstained from the royal beverages. However, the basis for Daniel's dietary experiment has been the subject of debate, and has been used by vegetarians, vegans, and prohibitionists alike to promote a variety of anti-meat, anti-dairy, and anti-alcohol agendas.

Defiled Kitchens and Defiling Fuel

Regardless, there is no evidence to suggest that Daniel's decisions were based on vegetarian, vegan, or abstinence convictions. Instead, there is every reason to surmise that Daniel's actions were a logical response to unclean and unkosher Babylonian dining norms, which were even predicted and prophesied through the prophet Ezekiel. Through vivid imagery of Ezekiel's prophetic example, God had described exactly what the Babylonian kitchens would be like.

> 'Eat the food as you would a barley cake; bake it in the sight of the people, using human excrement for fuel.' The Lord said, 'In this way the people of Israel will eat defiled food among the nations where I will drive them.' (Ezek. 4:12–13)

Ezekiel objected to God when presented with such a scenario, much like Daniel objected to the Babylonian chief official, and as Peter did to the voice in his vision more than six centuries later.

> Then I said, 'Not so, Sovereign Lord! I have never defiled myself. From my youth until now I have never eaten anything found dead or torn by wild animals. No unclean meat has ever entered my mouth.' (Ezek. 4:14)

Of course, in the case of Ezekiel, God did relent in response to his objection—allowing him to cook his food over cow dung instead of human defecation.[107] While the Ezekiel account might sound unusual in many ways, it does help establish or clarify a couple of interesting kosher principles.

Ezekiel's prophetic experience demonstrates the possible basis for Daniel's concerns, as well as offering an explanation for Paul's point in Romans—that "no food is unclean in itself" or more precisely, "no food can defile itself." However unpleasant it may be perceived per Western standards, grass-based cow manure is not deemed to be harmful for handling, heating, or cooking purposes according to Moses' law.[108] By nature and per Moses, a cow is a clean animal and so is everything inside of its unique system of cud-producing stomachs. Therefore, a cow, sheep, or goat lying in its own vegetation-comprised waste will not be rendered either "unclean" or "defiled"—regardless of the possible perceptions of vegans or vegetarians.[109]

In contrast, if the clean beef steak, lamb chop, or poultry comes in contact with the bodily fluid or defecation of either omnivores or carnivores, e.g., pigs, horses, rabbits, shellfish, humans, it becomes either "common" or "defiled," as in the case of Ezekiel's barley bread. There is every reason to believe that the royal Babylonian chefs did not distinguish between the clean and the unclean in their kitchens.

---

107 Ezekiel 4:15
108 Cow dung has been used as fuel for heating and cooking on every inhabited continent by dozens of cultures throughout the world.
109 Ezekiel 4:9-16

According to Moses, clay pots would become unclean and even impossible to clean once they were defiled with the carcass or "meat" of an unclean animal.[110] Given Daniel's great reverence and faithfulness, it stands to reason that he would not share dishes or counter space in the kitchen with the king's food—it is even likely that Daniel would object to sharing ovens with the Babylonians. Even if Daniel craved a kosher lamburger, he knew that his food would become defiled if it were cooking adjacent to unclean Babylonian meats, which might release wastes through residues and steam, as would burning unclean fuels such as human fecal matter. Thus it would be easiest, safest, most practical, and least offensive for Daniel to insist on a vegetable diet, at least until he could train the royal kitchen crew how to handle clean foods and dishes.

Defiled Grapes and Defiled Vineyards

In addition to avoiding foods defiled in the royal kitchen, Daniel also abstained from drinking the royal wine. Yet Daniel's reservations about wine were not coupled to abstinence mandates, as prohibitionists might infer without Scriptural evidence. To the contrary, Daniel knew that properly prepared wine or fermented drink was explicitly permitted by Moses[111] according to the Torah. Although Daniel may have been legitimately concerned about the storage vessels used for wine (wineskins may have been a pig stomach instead of a sheep or goat stomachs), Daniel may also have been concerned about the wine's ingredients.

While there is no obvious reference to the practice of crossbreeding crops in the book of Daniel, it is possible that the practice was commonplace in Babylon, even though it was forbidden by Moses.

Do not plant two kinds of seed[112] in your vineyard; if you

---

110 Leviticus 11:33

111 Deuteronomy 14:26

112 This commandment has modern implications relative to cross breeding of different species, i.e. genetically modified organisms (GMO).

do, not only the crops you plant but also the fruit of the vineyard will be defiled. (Deut. 22:9)

In yet another instance, Moses may have been describing the poisonous result of cross breeding as he described grapes of Sodom and Gomorrah, prior to the Israelite conquest of the land of Canaan.

> Their vine comes from the vine of Sodom and from the fields of Gomorrah. Their grapes are filled with poison, and their clusters with bitterness. Their wine is the venom of serpents, the deadly poison of cobras. (Deut. 32:32–33 NIV)

While it is credible that Babylon's wineries may have used grapes that were cross-pollinated with other crops, another and probable explanation exists. In fact, a number of Scriptures all point to narcotic wine additives. For example, the same Deuteronomy verse in the King James Version, like the original Hebrew and other prophets, alludes to the non-grape wine ingredients.

> "For their vine is of the vine of Sodom, and of the fields of Gomorrah: their grapes are grapes of gall, their clusters are bitter: Their wine is the poison of dragons, and the cruel venom of asps." (Deut. 32:32–33 KJV)

To liken the grapes[113] of Canaan to gall and bitterness is of particular significance. Gall[114] is repeatedly listed in the Bible in conjunction not only with bitterness[115] but with wormwood,[116] a bitter plant or root[117] capable of being distilled into an anise-flavored alcohol called absinthe. Such substances were not grown and harvested merely for flavoring.

---

113 Or more generically, fruit, עֵנָב, Strong's H6025
114 A poisonous (maybe poppy) plant or plant outgrowth, Strong's H7219
115 Strong's H4846
116 Strong's H3939
117 Artemisia absinthium

Defiled Wines and Defiled Minds

Potentially fermented or mixed with wine, wormwood has several uses—including that of a pain-numbing drug. Although used as an anesthetic by many cultures, the substance is also notorious for inviting hallucinations, is capable of attacking the nervous system, and is occasionally responsible for seizures or death. Although outlawed in many countries today, wormwood is still used in occult rituals, witchcraft, shamanism, and pagan religions to induce hallucinogenic effects.

With wormwood legends spanning all the way back to Eden, where it was said to be a product of the serpent's tail,[118] the substance was also known by Daniel's Babylon and Moses' Egypt. Relating wormwood's hallucinogenic effects to ancient idol worship, Moses warned Israel,

> Lest there should be among you man, or woman, or family, or tribe, whose heart turneth away this day from the Lord our God, to go and serve the gods of these nations; lest there should be among you a root that beareth gall and wormwood. (Deut. 29:18)

And just as the prophet Ezekiel predicted the defilement of solid foods in exile, so the prophet Jeremiah predicted Judah's use of wormwood for beverage in Babylon.

> Therefore thus saith the Lord of hosts, the God of Israel; Behold, I will feed them, even this people, with wormwood, and give them water of gall to drink. (Jer. 9:15)

Jeremiah elaborated on the implications of Babylonian wine consumption. Drawing connections between Jeremiah chapters 9 and 51, it is not difficult or far-reaching to connect Babylonian absinthe-wine mixtures with lunacy.

---

118 http://medicinalherbinfo.org/herbs/Wormwood.html

Babylon was a gold cup in the Lord's hand; she made the whole earth drunk. The nations drank her wine; therefore they have now gone mad. (Jer. 51:7)

Finally, Jeremiah lamented Jerusalem's fall and Judah's exile. Speaking on behalf of the people of the Judean kingdom, the prophet grieved,

He hath filled me with bitterness, he hath made me drunken with wormwood... Remembering mine affliction and my misery, the wormwood and the gall. (Lam. 3:15, 19 KJV)

Surely, being an educated young man, Daniel understood the cause and curse of the Babylonian exile; and he was discerning enough to rise above it.

During his crucifixion, Jesus also was offered wine mixed with gall or myrrh. He was in excruciating pain, nearing death. Two gospel accounts present this occurrence.

There they offered Jesus wine to drink, mixed with gall; but after tasting it, he refused to drink it. (Matt. 27:34)

Then they offered him wine mixed with myrrh, but he did not take it. (Mark 15:23)

Like the prophet Daniel, Jesus refused to allow himself to be defiled by gall or wormwood. Each man would uniquely avoid the cup of Babylon's judgment. Their third eye, otherwise known as the mind's eye—the locus of consciousness and place where the spirit is thought to unite with the body—would not be defiled; it would remain intact until the very moment that their spirits departed from their bodies. Neither Daniel nor Jesus would welcome the hallucinogenic "Green Fairy"[119] of insanity; they would not invite demons into their souls or share their bodies with evil and destructive spirits.

---

119 Absinthe is known for its distinct green appearance

Paul, Daniel, and a Guy Named Webster

Just as Daniel's dietary behavior cannot be understood without due consideration of context, neither can Paul's preaching be understood without the proper definition of simple terms. To their own harm, most Christian institutions within English-speaking cultures do not derive the meaning of the word 'food' from the Bible; instead, they formulate their beliefs on traditions and secular dictionary definitions. One dictionary, for example, defines food as "material, usually of plant or animal origin, that contains or consists of essential body nutrients, such as carbohydrates, fats, proteins, vitamins, or minerals, and is ingested and assimilated by an organism to produce energy, stimulate growth, and maintain life."[120] While such definitions may sound articulate, encompassing, and scientific, they are, in reality, oversimplified and morally benign. In accepting food as "anything ingested for caloric intake or bodily nourishment" in accordance with cultural norms, people fail to make distinction between animal and human diets, just as they overlook the moral components or religious aspects to food. Yet without considering the biblical aspects of food—moral and human—it is inevitable that Paul's writings to the Corinthians and Romans will be misunderstood.

Of course, Paul did not consult Webster as he wrote Romans or Corinthians any more than Moses did as he began writing the Torah. Yet this didn't deter anyone—from the patriarchs to the prophets—from arriving at a consistent and working definition of food. New Testament contributors found insight and inspiration in Moses' law, which came directly from God at Mount Sinai. As far as man is concerned, food should not be merely what the dictionary says it is; food was, is, and always will be exactly what an unchanging God says it is—ever since Genesis, as the next chapter illustrates.

While Paul was convinced that all food was clean,[121] he wasn't convinced that everything was created for food. Likewise, Peter didn't envision that everything was to be killed and eaten. Neither did Jesus

---

120 American Heritage Dictionary
121 Romans 14:20, 1 Timothy 4:1–5

declare all things to be food. And even in the event that Jesus did declare all animals to be clean food—which he did not—he would be legitimately branded as a false prophet and an apostate teacher in accordance with the words of the prophets Moses and Ezekiel.[122]

Defiled by Imagination

Is the defilement of food or drink merely a matter of imagination, and are unclean designations arbitrarily established in the mind of the beholder, as inferred by traditional religious institutions and implied by English Bible translations? Absolutely not.

Paul's letter to the Corinthians merely established that believers were not to eat at idolatrous festivals, or with other believers who were idolatrous hypocrites. Paul empowered believers with freedom and discretion, giving any Christian believer the latitude to eat with any unbelievers not engaged in idolatry. He also clarified that believers can eat food handled by idolatrous people, even if it passes through places engaged in pagan religious rituals, provided the food is eaten by the believer with thanksgiving to the one true God. Along with these clarifications, however, Paul admonished his audience to be especially careful when eating with new believers recovering from idolatry, lest they be inclined to revert back to paganism, some of them being still ignorant, superstitious, and of a "weak conscience." Obviously, new converts unfamiliar with Moses' writings would be unable to understand how foods became defiled, erroneously believing that idols had the power to defile food or make it unclean.

Likewise, Paul's letter to the Romans was written to a mixed audience, which included ignorant converts recovering from pagan influences. In Romans, Paul suggests that believers who were vegetarians or vegans as a result of moral or religious convictions were "weak in faith" or confused in their doctrine. Nevertheless, he also warned the more knowledgeable believers, who did eat meat derived from clean animals, against harshly abusing the new believers who failed to understand

---

122 Deuteronomy 13:4, Ezekiel 22:26

biblical dining principles and ordinances related to the defilement of meat. To this end, Paul reiterates that clean foods of any variety are not capable of becoming defiled or unclean in and of themselves, but that such foods could be defiled by mishandling. Likewise, the prophets (including Daniel, Ezekiel, and Moses) taught the same—foods could be defiled when contacting bodily fluids or unclean animal byproducts.

Daniel's account implicitly demonstrates that kitchens, butcher shops, and dishes that become defiled by processing unclean animals can defile clean food, and that not all living organisms are made for food. In addition to knowing that unclean food would corrupt the body, Jesus and Daniel also knew better than to defile the mind with poisonous drinks comprised of hallucinogenic substances. They used their God-given senses to make a right judgment and objected to consuming defiled 'food' as well as that which had the power to defile—as defined by Moses, not their personal imaginations.

Surely, Paul's works must be treated as progressive revelation built on complementary precepts as disclosed through earlier texts—not as unique anti-kosher revelations. By treating Paul's letters as instructions that embody kosher principles, one finds that they easily correlate with all earlier food and eating Bible texts, upholding simple cleanliness-godliness paradigms. Paul's instructions to "eat anything" are indisputably predicated on Genesis food definition—as described in the next chapter. In the same way, Paul's remarks that "no food is unclean in itself" and that "all food is clean" are contingent on Moses' original definitions pertaining to what is by nature *impure* and *unclean,* or what is by circumstance *defiled.*

Chapter 3 Notes

4

Red Meat, Green Meat, and the Genesis of Food

Then God said, "I give you every seed-bearing plant on the face of the whole earth and every tree that has fruit with seed in it. They will be yours for food. And to all the beasts of the earth... everything that has the breath of life in it—I give every green plant for food." And it was so."

—Gen. 1:29

And the Lord God commanded the man, "You are free to eat from any tree in the garden; but you must not eat from the tree of the knowledge of good and evil, for when you eat of it you will surely die."

—Gen. 2:16–17

Everything that lives and moves will be food for you. Just as I gave you the green plants, I now give you everything. But you must not eat meat that has its lifeblood still in it.

—Gen. 9:3

By using Moses' law as a key to decipher New Testament texts, many kosher eating principles that would otherwise remain lost in translation become plainly evident. Not surprisingly, the same principle also applies to understanding many other Old Testament accounts. Yet while Moses was instrumental in recording kosher principles in Bible texts, it is not difficult to see that kosher designations did not originate with Moses at Mount Sinai. In fact, kosher principles are introduced much earlier in Genesis; overt hints provided in Genesis even help show that kosher diets were introduced "In the Beginning."

Kindergarten Kosher

Much like Adam was appointed as the world's first taxonomist,[123] naming all of the animals, so too was Noah presented with a unique opportunity to become the world's greatest zoologist. Noah built an ark to preserve a multitude of animals many generations after Adam classified them, thus making him perhaps the foremost authority on animals that the world has ever known.

Of course, Noah's expertise in animal management can be deduced from the story of the flood, which is more than just a miraculous deliverance of beasts and birds. Noah had an enormous part to play, and he had a lot of work assigned to him in order that the task of redemption might be achieved. After being told about the upcoming flood, Noah designed, constructed, and stocked his ark to handle and feed all types of animals—including kosher ones. These responsibilities were delegated to Noah as God gave him the building plans, for God expressed no intentions of putting the animals into hibernation or

---

123 Genesis 2:19

another type of supernatural stasis; neither did he promise to feed the ship's passengers by manna from heaven.[124]

Given his responsibilities in preparing the ark, it is obvious that Noah would need to know what all of the animals ate and how much they ate—long before embarking on his historic voyage. Out of this necessity, Noah also had to know how to distinguish between clean and unclean animals long before Moses described them via quill and sheepskin, for they needed to be fed differently and loaded in different proportions.

Unfortunately for Noah, his logistical problems were multiplied in accordance with the number and types of animals that entered the ark. Contrary to popular Noachian cartoons and Sunday school projects that show animals trotting up the gangway in simple pairs, along with a few miscellaneous bird varieties perched on the rail or circling above the vessel, not all of the animal kinds boarded Noah's ark in sets of two. The Bible account tells a drastically different story; Noah brought both clean animals and birds aboard the ark in greater numbers, according to Genesis chapter 7. Unlike the unclean animals, which were admitted only in single pairs, the clean animals and birds were brought aboard in pairs of seven! Genesis is so literal in these details that even seven-year-old children should be able to understand it if they are invited to read the text for themselves. Even contemporary English translations of Genesis make unapologetic distinctions between the required numbers of clean and unclean animals.

> Take with you seven[125] of every kind of clean animal, a male and its mate, and two of every kind of unclean animal, a male and its mate, and also seven of every kind of bird, male and female, to keep their various kinds alive throughout the earth. (Gen. 7:2–3)

---

124 Genesis 6:21

125 The original Hebrew in Genesis 7:2 says there were "שבוע שבוע" (seven seven) animals, followed by "איש ואשתו" (a male and his female) which might be translated as "seven male and seven female" animals.

Despite the simplicity of this narrative, most media forms and paraphernalia portray a Noah's ark far from the Genesis text descriptions; from kindergarten toy sets to museum grade oil paintings, most depictions only show the animals loading in quantities of two, irrespective of type. Furthermore, they typically exclude familiar animals while including every exotic animal imaginable. It would seem that Noah's ark depictions are incomplete without pairs of zebras, elephants, lions, tigers, hippos, horses, panda bears, gorillas, monkeys, kangaroos, parrots, flamingos, penguins, ostriches, camels, snakes, crocodiles, turtles, and lizards. However, animal varieties from Old McDonald's farm are few and far between—while those from Tarzan's jungle are present in disproportionate excess.

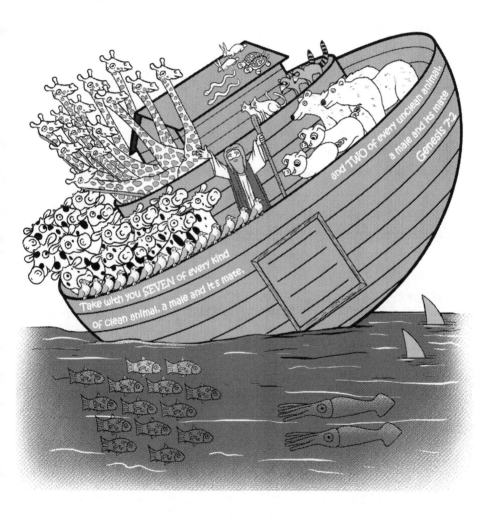

Old McNoah Had an Ark, E-I-E-I-O

Sadly, after gleaning their theology from Noah's ark merchandise and assorted toy sets, children are more likely to envision pairs of unicorns and purple ponies boarding the ark than a diverse collection of farm animals in their proper proportion. Still less exciting domesticated animals, such as cows, sheep, goats, ducks, and doves seem to be excluded—almost deliberately—from the toy collections and artwork. If not for exotic mammals like antelope, there might be no clean animals aboard some of the imaginary arks. From these images, children must be forced to assume that Noah's animals came from remote places like Africa, Asia, the Amazon rainforest, or even the Galapagos Islands, while the ark lacked access to ordinary farm animals. Also, for reasons unexplained, wild and clean North American animals, such as buffalo, moose, and deer seem to miss the boat on most occasions as well— unless the reindeer figures are misplaced. While exotic giraffes, with heads towering above the rest of the animals, always find their way onto the ark, they tend to be in short supply. Giraffes are never presented in sevens as the clean, split-hoofed, cud-chewing mammals that they are; they are seen as lone couples boarding along with other foreign species of the Serengeti. If the Genesis texts were taken seriously, a small herd of fourteen giraffes would always stand out above two elephants[126]— wherever the ark is pictured!

Whether they are of the domesticated or wild variety, the overall shortage of clean animals on Noah's ark is disconcerting. The clean versus unclean animal count in the ark story may sound like a trivial detail, but the tendency to misrepresent animal proportions may speak volumes. Not only does the misrepresentation undermine the magnificence of Noah's narrative, it detracts profoundly from kosher causes.

---

126 Genesis 6:19 indicates that just two unclean animals (Strong's 8147, שנים, shenayim or "couples") were to be boarded, describing the pair as a gender matched set. The gender-matched pairs are also described in Genesis 7:8-9, where שנים שנים is describing the couples of clean animals boarding the ark along with couples of unclean animals.

The shortage of clean ark animals in contrast to the surplus of unclean animals presents more questions than answers. Do people portray an ark full of unclean animals as a matter of preference? How could so many coloring books, toy sets, and Sunday school classes present the story wrongly—and for so long? Is this a conspiracy concocted by toy companies, with the objective of reducing the piece count for purposes of economy? Could it be too exhausting for families to pick up playrooms if proper proportions of Noah's clean animals clutter the floor? Or is it just too hard to teach young children how to count seven pairs? Surely, the myth of "three wise men riding on camels"[127] at Christmas pales in comparison and in its implications! If nothing else, the prevalence of incomplete Noah's ark sets and artwork testifies to the prominence of dogma, in which poor graphic media perpetuates ignorance, triumphing over original texts.

Wild Instinct Suspension

The automatic gathering of the animals prior to the flood is another detail of the Noah's account that hints to kosher animal categories already present prior to the flood. In particular, the normal instincts of wild animals—as opposed to kosher ones—is described as being divinely transformed or suspended at the time of the flood. Prior to the flood, Genesis describes a supernatural ingathering of wild animal pairs.

> You are to bring into the ark two of all living creatures, male and female, to keep them alive with you. Two of every kind of bird, of every kind of animal and of every kind of creature that moves along the ground will come to you to be kept alive. (Gen. 6:19-20)

Needless to say, a miraculously cooperative wild animal population would save Noah a great deal of difficulty in loading his ark. This being the case, perhaps the ark cartoons do convey an element of truth. They

---

127 The texts introduce three types of gifts, but not three men, ref. Matthew 2:1.

depict wild animals cooperatively mustering before the ark in a single file line; even the animals that are otherwise ferocious appear friendly, such as lions, tigers, and bears, smiling ear to ear beside Noah—with no intention of eating him! Yet when the miracle ark ride was over, the wild animals' special disposition and relationship of necessity seems to come to an end. Immediately after the flood as Noah and his sons were blessed, they were told that "fear and dread" would return to the animals.[128] Thus, the change and restoration of animal behavior could be perceived as described below.

Wild animals with fear of man
(before the flood)
↓
Wild animals not hostile toward man
(during time of the ark)
↓
Wild animals with fear of man
(after the flood)

It is also of note that the suspension of wild animal behavior described in the Genesis text cited above seems to have applied only to the animal pairs of two—appearing to correspond with the unclean varieties. However, there is good reason to believe that the wild instinct suspension described above did not apply to the clean animals.

Clean 'Livestock' for Food

Immediately after informing Noah about the pairs of wild animals that would arrive before the flood, God also told Noah about his responsibility in gathering "food" for his animal cargo.

---

128 Genesis 9:2

You are to take every kind of food that is to be eaten and store it away[129] as food for you and for them. (Gen. 6:21)

Beginning an entire week before the flood, Noah and family would finally begin boarding the ark along with all types of animals. In contrast with the unclean animals that showed up for the occasion with their wild instincts suspended, it is logical to surmise that Noah had already collected the multitude of clean animals that would be used to feed the animals of the unclean variety. To this point, it would appear that Noah could also simply 'take' the clean animals on board, with no divine prodding or assembly mentioned in the text.

The Lord then said to Noah, "Go into the ark, you and your whole family, because I have found you righteous in this generation. Take with you seven of every kind of clean animal, a male and its mate..." (Gen. 7: 1–2)

Without making allusion to a miraculous clean animal gathering of seven pairs prior to this point,[130] and giving specific direction for Noah to collect "food" in verses prior, these latter verses might suggest that the clean animals were taken aboard as "food" by Noah. Of greater significance, it also suggests that the clean animals were already under the control of Noah's family, likely stored in cages or stables as livestock, readily available for the taking just before boarding. Thus, it is evident that Noah and his sons were well prepared to enjoy kosher meat while on the ark, relying on their surplus clean animal cargo in part for

---

129 The Hebrew word for "store it away" is better translated as "collect" or "gather" (אסף, 'âsaph, Strong's H622), which is closely related to the Hebrew word for "add" or "increase," (יסף, yâsaph, Strong's H3254), which is used in context of bearing offspring.

130 The text might also allow for clean pairs to arrive via Genesis 6:19-20, with Noah assuming the responsibility of increasing the herd sizes per Genesis 6:21-22, such that he arrived at 7 pairs of clean animals at Genesis 7:2.

food.[131] This "clean-livestock-for-food" interpretation best explains the otherwise grossly disproportionate 7-to-1 ratio between the animal types, and the need for more clean animals.[132] Unclean animals are often carnivorous by design, and only a single pair of clean animals was really required to preserve the species and repopulate the planet. Therefore, if not loaded for the exclusive purpose of food, during and after the flood, there is no other viable explanation accounting for the offset numbers.[133]

Furthermore, the Scriptures indicate that following the flood, the ark landed with surplus clean animals, and that Noah and his sons used a fraction of those animals for sacrifices. The Genesis account states,

> Then Noah built an altar to the Lord and, taking some of all the clean animals and clean birds, he sacrificed burnt offerings on it. (Gen. 8:20)

Per the text, it is legitimate to assume that Noah still had a surplus of clean animals after the ark and after offering the sacrifice.[134] Without a doubt, the remaining clean animals would continue to serve as food

---

131 Human dietary needs would be a fraction of Noah's clean animal cargo. A single cow can produce hundreds of pounds of beef, which Noah and family may have shared with unclean animals, and which would be occasionally slaughtered for the sake of unclean animal feed.

132 The 7 to 1 ratio also seems to be consistent with the ark's human cargo. Noah brought 3 sons, and each man on the ark had a wife. However, terminology from Leviticus 18:7 suggests that Ham had a forbidden sexual relationship with Noah's wife in Genesis 9:22, producing Canaan. Thus, Noah cursed Canaan in Genesis 9:25, much like Moses warranted the excommunication of the inbred in Deuteronomy 22:30-23:2. Thus, Ham might be considered as the lone unclean and impure passenger on board the ark relative to the 7 perfect or pure family members.

133 Unclean carnivorous mammals often reproduce in larger litters than do clean mammal varieties, thus they would need a head start in repopulating the planet, and hence the 7-to-1 ratio.

134 Even if only a single clean animal of each variety was offered, slaughtering and butchering animals of every clean variety as the text describes would take days; therefore it is impractical to infer that the majority of the seven clean pairs were boarded exclusively for the sake of sacrifice.

after the flood—both for the people and for the many unclean animal species that depended on a carnivorous diet.

Blessed to Eat—Again

Logic, of course, would preclude Noah and sons from using any endangered species for food, such as one of the last of a breeding pair of unclean animals, like pigs, horses, lions, or turtles—especially after going through such drama to save all of the animal types from extinction in a catastrophic global flood. Immediately following the clean animal sacrifice, God blessed Noah and kin, saying,

> Be fruitful and increase in number and fill the earth. The fear and dread of you will fall upon all the beasts of the earth and all the birds of the air, upon every creature that moves along the ground, and upon all the fish of the sea; they are given into your hands. Everything that lives and moves will be food for you. Just as I gave you the green plants, I now give you everything. But you must not eat meat that has its lifeblood still in it. (Gen. 9:1–4 NIV)

At the point of this blessing, the animals' fear of man would return to them, while Noah and kin would transform from earthy, pre-flood vegans to flesh-craving, post-flood omnivores—at least as many religious traditions would have it. Per popular religious dogma and dispensational interpretations, Noah's generation was the first to be granted the luxury of eating "everything" set before them.

But did God really expand the definition of food as Adam and Eve knew it, blessing Noah and his family differently after they disembarked from the ark? Surely it is unsound to think that God would allow Noah and sons to declare open season on any beast exiting the ark, since this "all animals for food" view might implicate Noah and his family in hunting dinosaurs to extinction—while they still had clean animals to spare for food! Was this post-flood age truly a new era, like that of Peter, with God essentially saying, "Get out, Noah; kill, and eat!"?

Extra Dispensational Gifts

Per the Genesis 9 citation above, the account of Noah's blessing reads as if God endowed man with two different diets—an omnivore one under Noah after the flood, and an earlier vegetarian one under Adam. However, the New International Version begins to appear suspicious when compared to older translations, like the one cited below.

> Every moving thing that liveth shall be meat for you; even
> as the green herb <u>have I given</u> you all things. (Gen. 9:3 KJV)

Likewise, in the original Hebrew, the text makes but a single reference to "giving."

9:3	כָּל	-	רֶמֶשׂ		אֲשֶׁר	הוּא - חַי		לָכֶם
	kl	-	rmsh		ashr	eua - chi		l·km
	every-of		moving-animal		which	he	life	to·you (p)

יִהְיֶה		לְאָכְלָה	כְּיֶרֶק		עֵשֶׂב		נָתַתִּי
ieie		l·akle	k·irq		oshb		nththi
he-is-becoming		for·food	as·greens		herbage		I-give

לָכֶם		אֵת - כָּל		:
l·km		ath - kl		:
to·you (p)	»	all		

(Gen. 9:3 ISA)

In the original Hebrew, as well as in the King James Version, verse 3 has but one occurrence of נתתי[135] or "I give," or "I have given," which, if alluding to Adam and Eve's blessing—where man was first given green things to eat—might also be interpreted in the past tense form.

---

135 From Strong's H5414, נתן (nâthan), to give

Doubling the Hebrew gave/give verb count and juxtaposing the two resulting English verbs into past and present tenses—as the NIV citation does on page 99—gives the account a grossly exaggerated and strong dispensational slant. Likewise, the NIV text adds to the confusion by including an extra present-tense adverb, i.e., "I *now* give" to further bolster the dispensational distinction between past and present eras. In slight contrast, the single occurrence in the King James text uses the passive "have I given" phrase, which inclines a reader to associate the event with Noah, assuming a recent past-tense rendering of the verb phrase. But how does this affect the meaning of the message, and which view is correct?

The Vegans of Eden

To resolve this give/gave verb tense question in Noah's account, the details of both Adam's and Noah's blessings must be examined and compared. First introducing the permissive fruits-and-vegetables dietary statements for Adam and Eve, the blessing of Genesis 1 is cited below.

> God blessed them and said to them, "Be fruitful and increase in number; fill the earth and subdue it. Rule over the fish of the sea and the birds of the air and over every living creature that moves on the ground."
>
> Then God said, "I give you every seed-bearing plant on the face of the whole earth and every tree that has fruit with seed in it. They will be yours for food.
>
> "And to all the beasts of the earth and all the birds of the air and all the creatures that move on the ground—everything that has the breath of life in it—I give every green plant for food." And it was so. (Gen. 1:28–30 NIV)

According to the contemporary translation above and nearly every English interpretation of this Genesis text, humanity was originally commissioned through Adam and Eve to eat as vegans. From that standpoint, it is logical to infer that God would recall the earlier blessing of plants and fruits given to Adam and Eve as he blessed Noah after the flood.

Vegan Animal Kingdom Anomalies

Adding a bizarre twist to the story, English translations of Genesis 1 text present all of the animals as having similar green plant-based diets. They are even translated as if God disallowed any animal to eat fruit—or as if God created mammals capable of multiplication without mothers' mammary glands. Even the King James Version seems to reinforce the traditional views of Eden as a vegan animal kingdom.

> And to every beast of the earth, and to every fowl of the air, and to every thing that creepeth upon the earth, wherein *there is* life, *I have given* every green herb for meat:[136] and it was so. (Gen. 1: 30 KJV)

However prominent such Genesis 1 interpretations may be, the vegan animal kingdom views implied by English translations present a number of logical conflicts. For example, why would God speak to man in the preceding verse, giving mankind a blessing of multiplication, and a blessing of dominion, and then immediately afterward begin to issue instructions for animal diets? Surely, it is nothing less than strange for God to grant humans dominion over the animal kingdom, while then articulating the diet of the entire animal kingdom in the very next breath. Since animals far outnumber mankind, it's not as if Adam and Eve would be able to exercise their dominion by managing diets of all of the animals. Moreover, they would not need to oversee animal diets, as animals were instilled with instincts and appetites to govern their behavior, and they were endowed with the apparatus

---

136 The KJV was written four centuries ago, when the English term "meat" generically referred to food, not exclusively to food derived from animal flesh, as it does today.

and aptitudes to acquire and process whatever food is fitting for them. Clearly, governing over animal diets or feeding every living species hardly qualifies as humanity having dominion over the animals. To the contrary, Adam and Eve were assigned to work on a garden plot, not in a free-range petting zoo created for the sake of animal feeding. God did not establish Eden as a welfare state for the sake of animal dependency. Such an arrangement would be one of human servitude, not of human dominion.

Also, there's the matter of timing in the Genesis account as it might pertain to an exaggerated human dominion over the animals. Would God expect the birds and fish created on day five to go hungry waiting for food until man arrived on day six?[137] Did animals on day five need to wait another day until God finished creating and blessing the balance of the animal kingdom before they began to eat the green herbs?

Finally, if the entire animal kingdom was created vegan, why would God include the birds while excluding the fish from his vegan animal kingdom as listed in verse 30? Surely, God would not be so careless as to create the waters without green plants or simple algae to feed the aquatic life!

Generous Translators and Translation Addendum

Strangely enough, to resolve all the inconsistencies arising from vegan animal kingdom views of Genesis 1 is to also resolve the open questions emerging from Noah's confusing omnivore diet blessing in Genesis 9; the exact same error confounding the translation of Noah's dietary blessing is repeated in the case of Adam's dietary blessing. In comparing the Hebrew text below to traditional English versions, it is clear that the translators generously "gave" or interjected an extra and presumptuous "I give" (נתתי) verb to verse 30, presuming that the verb from verse 29 may be doubled and inserted into the next verse for clarity and without ill effect. Once again, for the reader's edification, the word-for-word interlinear Hebrew text is provided below.

---

137 Genesis 1:22

1:29 וַיֹּאמֶר הִנֵּה אֱלֹהִים נָתַתִּי
u·iamr aleim ene nththi
and·he-is-saying Elohim behold! I-give

לָכֶם אֵת ־ כָּל ־ עֵשֶׂב ־ זֹרֵעַ זֶרַע
l·km ath - kl - oshb zro zro
to·you⁽ᴾ⁾ » every-of herbage seeding seed

אֲשֶׁר עַל ־ פְּנֵי כָל ־ הָאָרֶץ וְאֵת ־
ashr ol - phni kl - e·artz u·ath -
which on surfaces-of all-of the·earth and·»

כָּל ־ הָעֵץ אֲשֶׁר ־ בּוֹ פְרִי ־ עֵץ
kl - e·otz ashr - b·u phri - otz
every-of the·tree which in·him fruit-of tree

לְאָכְלָה : יִהְיֶה לָכֶם זֶרַע זֹרֵעַ
l·akle : ieie l·km zro zro
for·food : he-is-becoming for·you⁽ᴾ⁾ seed seeding

1:30 עוֹף ־ וּלְכָל ־ הָאָרֶץ חַיַּת ־ וּלְכָל
u·l·kl - ouph e·artz u·l·kl - chith
and·for·every-of flyer-of the·land animal-of and·for·every-of

עַל ־ רוֹמֵשׂ וּלְכֹל הַשָּׁמַיִם
ol - rumsh u·l·kl e·shmim
on moving-animal and·for·every-of the·heavens

כָּל ־ אֵת ־ חַיָּה נֶפֶשׁ בּוֹ ־ אֲשֶׁר הָאָרֶץ
ath - kl - chie nphsh b·u - ashr e·artz
every-of » living soul in·him which the·land

כֵּן ־ : וַיְהִי לְאָכְלָה עֵשֶׂב יֶרֶק
kn - : u·iei l·akle oshb irq
so - : and·he-is-becoming for·food herbage green

(Gen. 1:29–30 ISA)

By not adding a second נתתי (I give) verb to verse 30, it is both simple and logical to derive a notably different translation from the Hebrew text, as suggested by the interlinear English text cited above. Moreover, by considering alternate definitions from *Strong's Concordance* in place of certain versatile Hebrew words, a unique and more informative translation is possible, as shown below.

> And God says, behold, I have given to you each plant generating seed which is on the face of the whole earth and each tree which in its tree fruit generates seed—for you it is existing for food; and for each animal of the earth, and for each bird of the heavens, and for each moving animal on the earth—which in him *there is* a soul sustained by all green plants—for *your* food it is therefore existing. (Gen. 1:29-30 Author's Translation)

Given that the original Hebrew language does not include punctuation, the possibility for a different sentence structure and word association becomes evident when an extra נתתי (I give) verb is not interjected into verse 30. To better illustrate this, Tables 1a-2b are provided to allow for side-by-side translation comparison.

TABLE 1A—GENESIS 1:29 TRANSLATIONS: KOSHER VARIATIONS

Verse 29 by Section	Original Hebrew	Author's Translation	ISA Interlinear Translation
God declares to give to people	ויאמר	and he is saying	and he is saying
	אלהים	God	Elohim
	הנה	behold	behold
	נתתי	I have given	I give
	לכם	to you	to you
seeded veggies	את-כל	each	every
	עשׂב	plant	herb
	זרע	generating	seeding
	זרע	seed	seed
	אשׁר	which is	which
	על-פני	on the face (of)	on surface
	כל-הארץ	the whole earth	all of the earth
and seeded fruits from trees	ואת-כל	and each	and every
	העץ	tree	tree
	אשׁר-בו	which in its	which in him
	פרי-עץ	tree fruit	fruit of tree
	זרע	generates	seeding
	זרע	seed	seed
for the ongoing purpose of human food it is	לכם	for you	for you
	יהיה[138]	it is being	he is becoming
	לאכלה	for food	for food

to v30

---

138 The verb יהיה (from Strong's H1961, hâyâh, meaning "to be") is presented in an imperfect form, referring to an ongoing state of existence, and not alluding to a beginning, as implied by the interlinear "becoming" text; neither should the verb be rendered as a "shall" permissive mandate or a "will" predictive permissive statement, as presented in popular English translations (see Table 2a).

TABLE 2A— GENESIS 1:29 TRANSLATIONS: VEGAN VARIATIONS

Verse 29 by Section		Original Hebrew	King James Version	New International Version
God declares to give		ויאמר	and said	then said
		אלהים	God	God
		הנה	behold	
		נתתי	I have given	I give
to people		לכם	you	you
	seeded veggies	את-כל	every	every
		עשׂב	herb	plant
		זרע	bearing	seed-
		זרע	seed	bearing
		אשׁר	which is	
		על-פני	upon the face of	on the face of
veggies and fruits		כל-הארץ	all the earth	the whole earth
	and seeded fruits from trees	ואת-כל	and every	and every
		העץ	tree	tree
		אשׁר-בו	in the which is the	that has
		פרי-עץ	fruit of a tree	fruit
		זרע	yielding	
		זרע	seed	with seed in it
prescribing it as future human food		לכם	to you	yours
		יהיה	it shall be	they will be
		לאכלה	for meat	for food

TABLE 1B— GENESIS 1:30 TRANSLATIONS: KOSHER VARIATIONS

Verse 30 by Section			Original Hebrew	Author's Translation	ISA Interlinear Translation
and for each	beast		ולכל	and for each	and for every of
			חית	animal of	animal of
			הארץ	the earth	the land
	bird		ולכל	and for each	and for every of
			עוף	bird of	flyer of
			השמים	the heavens	the heavens
animal	bug		ולכל	and for each	and for every of
			רומש	moving animal	moving animal
having			על-הארץ	on the earth	on the land
in it a soul	whose soul lives by greens		אשר-בו	which is in him	which in him
living by all			נפש	a soul	soul
green foliage			חיה[139]	living by	living
			את-כל[140]	all	every of
			ירק	green	green
			עשב	plants	herbage
for the ongoing purpose of (human) food it is			לאכלה	for (your) food	for food
			ויהי[141]	it is being	he is becoming
			כן	therefore	so

(arrow) from v29

---

139 In conventional translations of Genesis 1:30, the English pronoun and verb "I give" (equivalent to נתתי) is added by translators. In so doing, the את ('êth, Strong's H853) is assumed to designate green herbs as the direct object (i.e., the gift from God) of the inferred verb, with animals assumed to be the indirect object (i.e., the gift recipients).

140 Unlike verse 29, verse 30 associates no pronoun with the prepositional phrase "for food" or לאכלה, thus leaving the reader open to decide to which noun the term should be applied.

141 Like the verb יהיה as discussed in verse 29 notes, ויהי is written in an imperfect form and should not be rendered in a completed or "was" past tense form. In other words, ויהי should not be treated as a mere affirmation of events that transpired.

TABLE 2B— GENESIS 1:30 TRANSLATIONS: VEGAN VARIATIONS

Verse 30 by Section		Original Hebrew	King James Version	New International Version
and to	beasts	ולכל	and to every	and to all
		חית	beast of	the beasts of
		הארץ	the earth	the earth
animals	birds	ולכל	and to every	and all
		עוף	fowl of	the birds of
		השמים	the air	the air
that are living	bugs	ולכל	and to every	and all the
		רומש	thing that creepeth	creatures that move
		על-הארץ	upon the earth	on the ground
"God gives"	qualified as	אשר-בו	wherein there is	everything that has the
	living	נפש		breath of
		חיה	life	life in it
green plants	"given"	----------142	*I have given*	*I give*
for (their) food	all green plants	את-כל	every	every
		ירק	green	green
		עשב	herb	plant
		לאכלה143	for meat	for food
in the past.		ויהי144	and it was	and it was
		כן	so	so

142 Given that חיה (châyâh, Strong's H2421) is acting as a verb meaning "live" or "sustain" instead of an adjective (Strong's H2416) qualifying animal souls, translator interjection of the verse 29 verb/pronoun נתתי (I gave) into verse 30 is unwarranted.

143 With recipients of God's gifts being human and חיה acting as a verb, the את does not designate כל ירק עשב as a gift or exclusive animal diet; rather the phrase אשר בו נפש חיה (which is its soul sustained) is expanded with the את to encompass כל ירק עשב (all green plants), thus the animal's soul or נפש is qualified.

144 If beasts, birds, and bugs are not treated as objects of the verb נתתי (I gave) from verse 29, animals might be rendered as subjects relating to the verb ויהי. Thus, animal subjects have a purpose (i.e., "being for food"), joined casually (i.e., "therefore") with condition (i.e., "green soul"). Left alone, verse 30 suggests this, "And for every beast, bird, and bug [with a soul sustained by green plants], for food it exists therefore."

While some of the particular words used in translations above might be subject to scrutiny or debate, the two basic views of the translations as contrasted in Tables 1a, 1b, 2a and 2b might be simplified even further, as shown in Figure 1 below.

FIGURE 1—GENESIS 1 FOOD TRANSLATION COMPARISON

Genesis 1:29-30 Simplified Literal (i.e., Interlinear/Kosher) View

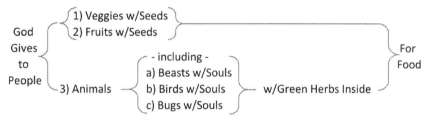

Genesis 1:29-30 Simplified Traditional (i.e., KJV/NIV/Vegan) View

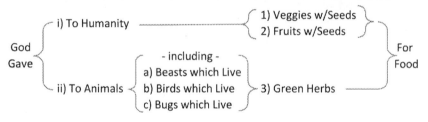

Although both views come from the same text and ultimately present the same nouns, the two views differ drastically with respect to the blessing's perceived audience, perceived gifts, and perceived recipients. Thus, they differ in the qualification of objects, which are modified by different verbs, prepositions, and nouns.

Green Herb Gifts versus Green Herb Qualifications

How ought this complex string of compound conditions be understood? Were the "green herbs" intended to be "gifts" for the animals alone, or do the "green herbs" instead qualify animal types by their stomach contents or energy source, thereby indicating which types are suitable for human consumption? Surely, the answers to such questions about Eden's food blessing have far-reaching implications, ranging from a vegan animal kingdom to an eternal kosher worldview.

While it may be rather bold—and even seem blasphemous—to criticize or even question assumptions driving popular English Bible translations, including those which have stood unchallenged within the Christian church for four centuries, it's not as if the basis for doing so is trivial. To the contrary, the original Genesis language, the surrounding context, latter parallel scriptural teachings, laws of biology, logic, and the health and well being of humanity seem to collectively demand nothing less!

As introduced in pages prior, there are numerous logical problems, like those of audience, dominion, instinct, chronology, and language, which inherently undermine the traditional "vegan blessing" views. In Genesis 1, God spoke a blessing to humanity, declaring human dominion over animals, having created them hungry and with instincts and appetites the day before the blessing was uttered. God spoke deliberately and coherently, to a species created with ears to hear, with an intellect capable of processing complex language, and the memory to retain the instructions; and God spoke each word for a human purpose. Being an omniscient being, it only stands to reason that God would put forth rational instructions to rational creatures; he did not create creatures with "dead souls", and did not need to limit the green food to animals with "living souls" when it is impossible for "dead souls" to eat. Likewise, God would hardly declare human food in the future tense saying "it will be for food", while speaking of animal food in the past tense, saying, "for food it was so" to an animal audience of limited cognitive potential for the sake of posterity.

Finally, a vegan Genesis worldview would seem to put either the Bible record or God's competency at stake. After all, it is written that when God created all life forms, the creation was "good". Furthermore, God "created everything according to its kind". Yet the Bible never seems to go on record saying that God "modified everything according to another kind", as a Genesis 1 vegan view implicitly demands. To suggest that there was a transformation between animal types is an argument from silence.

Leviticus in Genesis

Further supporting an eternal kosher worldview, it is of note that the animal "kinds" that were created in Genesis 1 coincided with the four "kinds" of animals described later in Moses' law, as introduced back in chapter 2. According to Leviticus 11, animals acceptable to eat also consist of four basic types:

✓ Land mammals—only split-hoofed and cud-chewing
✓ Crawling things—only joint-legged, hopping insects[145]
✓ Flying things—no birds of prey or scavenging birds
✓ Marine creatures—only scaled and finned fish

While marine animals are casually omitted from Genesis 1:29-30, the verses do nevertheless establish the first overarching kosher principle, namely, that *the clean eat green*! In the blessing of Eden, God was not saying that every animal in creation is required to graze on green plants.[146] He was saying that any air-breathing animals that exclusively eat green plants[147] were given to humanity as kosher to eat—from head to hoof. God wasn't limiting man to a diet of beans and apples—either temporarily or eternally, while allocating only green grasses to animals. In the beginning, God created complex ecosystems, which included all kinds of interdependent species. God didn't create a horse that didn't love apples[148], force the fruit bat to eat "green herbs" for a limited period, or introduce the vampire bat at a later time. God didn't expect the

---

145 e.g., locusts, grasshoppers, etc.
146 Fish are blessed to multiply in a prior verse, but their diet is not listed in the text.
147 Kosher mammals (e.g., cows and goats), unlike other herbivore animals (e.g., horses) can get sick and die from ingesting fruits and seeds (e.g., apples) due to stomach boating or seed toxins.
148 Seeded fruits/plants were not allotted to animals in Genesis 1:30.

dolphin to starve to death or demand that birds fast for a day because he was sloppy in the timing or scope of his Genesis green food blessing. Likewise, there is no evidence to demonstrate that the great white shark was equipped or directed to dine on plumes of ocean algae prior to Adam and Eve's misbehavior.

Humanity could not be fruitful, multiply, or have the dominion over the entire earth as described in Genesis 1:28 without being offered the nourishment to do so; and nourishment for people is exactly what God fully "gave" to all humanity, according to Genesis 1 verses 29 and 30.

Returning to Noah after Adam

Yet even after parsing out misleading translation addenda and restoring the original meaning to the blessings of Genesis, there are still more proofs testifying to a kosher blessing for the Noachian world. For example, it is undisputed that God specifically gave humanity seeded vegetables (עשב זרע זרע)[149] and seeded fruit from trees (פרי-עץ זרע זרע) to eat per Adam's blessing in Genesis 1, as shown on pages 101-110. Yet in comparing this to Noah's blessing on page 100, it is clear that God instead referred to green foliage (ירק עשב)[150] in the Genesis 9 Hebrew text. Thus, to assume from Noah's Genesis 9 blessing that Adam's diet was originally green herbs or foliage (ירק עשב) is to suggest that God only gave Adam green foliage to graze on—the same term to describe animal feed—instead of fruits and vegetables, as stated in Genesis 1. Because the blessing of Noah does not mention plants or fruits of a seeded variety for man, it is not reasonable to infer that God was comparing Noah's new omnivore animal diet upgrade with Adam's primitive vegan diet.

In addition to erroneous vegetation association and the exaggeration of the give/gave verb count and verb tense, the English translations are further distorted as a result of the misinterpretation of a single

---

149 Strong's H6212, H2232, and H2233
150 Strong's H6212 and H3418

preposition in Noah's blessing. By ignoring or misappropriating a single "כ", which is a prepositional prefix preceding the green herbs (כירק עשב), English translations (such as the NIV citation on page 99) fail to properly convey the original language's qualification or causality. Rather than using the preposition to qualify the herbs, the NIV seems to use the "just as" preposition to qualify the "I gave" verb instead. However, if the "according to" preposition is properly incorporated in the translation, the kosher animal diet connections—as originally revealed in Genesis 1—are found to be reiterated in Noah's Genesis 9 food blessing.[151]

> Every moving thing which lives for you, it will be for food *according to* the green herbs; I gave to you every such thing. (Gen. 9:3 AHT)[152]

Failing to recognize the 'grazing herbivore' principle and the contrasting vegetation types discussed in Genesis 1 and 9, even the popular King James Version inserts an "as" in the place of the "כ" preposition, thereby likening the edible animal types to the green foliage used for animal feed instead of conveying causality or qualification. While this preposition translation is listed as an equally permissible option per Strong's Concordance,[153] the context clearly dictates the use of "according to" over an "as" in the place of the "כ" preposition, for "according to" better conveys the conditional relationship between human dietary laws and edible animal types based on animal food

---

151 This literal vegan animal diet interpretation of the Genesis 1 and 9 texts may help explain Exodus 23:19, Exodus 34:26, and Deuteronomy 14:21, which prohibit a young calf or kid being "ripened" (בשל, bâshal, Strong's H1310) or growing on the milk of its mother. Thus, young animals may not be considered fit for human consumption as they are milk-fed, e.g., veal or young lamb. This may also correspond with texts prescribing 4 day period of separation of Passover lambs per Exodus 12:3-6.

152 Author's translation

153 Assuming Strong's H3644 (כמו, kâmô) is to be exchanged for the preposition "כ", terms such as "when" or "according to" may be preferable English substitutes, as employed in the KJV translations of Genesis 6:22, Genesis 24:30, and Genesis 29:13.

types.[154] After all, to say that "it will be food *as* (or *like*) the green herbs" upholds the old "you are what you eat" adage if applied to grazing animals, but it does not work for people who are not grazing on green herbs or foliage—as originally intended for animal feed.

Therefore, after comparing the blessings of Adam and Noah in Genesis chapters 1 and 9, it should be apparent that the combined blessing accounts do not lend themselves to dispensational interpretation; God's kosher animal gifting to humanity was repeated to Noah in a perfect and eternal tense. In the new post-flood beginning, Noah was told essentially the same things[155] as Adam,[156] that man was to be fruitful and multiply, that man had dominion over the animals, and that only green-eating varieties of animals were acceptable for man's food.[157]

Lifeblood versus Souls of Blood

The same animal diet and physiology arguments can also be used to disqualify certain animal types as food per the next verse of Noah's blessing.

But you must not eat meat that has its lifeblood still in it. (Gen. 9:4)

However, in order to entertain arguments of animal diets and

---

154 In the event that the preposition "כ" might be an abbreviated form of Strong's H3588 (כִּי, kîy), words conveying stronger conditional or causal relationships, such as "because," "when," "if," or "since," may alternatively be considered in translation.
155 Genesis 9:3
156 Another possible interpretation of the blessing is that Noah was permitted to resume his omnivorous kosher diet during his post-flood blessing, although there is no text indicating that Noah was given any restrictions on carnivorous dining before boarding the ark.
157 The same blessings, multiplication, food, and dominion are described per Genesis 1:28–30 and 9:1–3. It is reasonable to infer that man's dominion over animals was reiterated to Noah given man's participation in the pre-flood corruption of animals per Genesis 6:12; see also Enoch 7.

physiology within verse 4, it becomes essential to examine the text in the original Hebrew.

9:4   אַךְ -   בָּשָׂר   בְּנַפְשׁוֹ   דָמוֹ

```
     ak  -  bshr   b·nphsh·u        dm·u
     yea    flesh  in·soul-of·him   blood-of·him
```

לֹא   תֹאכֵלוּ :

```
la     thaklu :
not    you(p)-shall-eat
```

(Gen. 9:4 ISA)

While the Hebrew in the verse above contains three separate pronouns, the association of the pronouns becomes a matter of prerogative for the reader or translator. In most translations, the pronoun (denoted by "ו" or vav) in בנפשו and דמו is assumed to refer only to the same animal. However, in recognizing how animal diets and animal physiology are used to qualify animals that are suitable for human consumption, as is consistent with Bible texts,[158] it becomes apparent that the two Hebrew "ו" (vav) pronouns can concurrently refer to two different animals instead of the same one.[159] In other words, if two references to "him" that the text includes are not tied to other common nouns in adjacent texts, the reference to "him" could be construed as ambiguous; therefore, the second pronoun appended to the term דמו or "blood of him" might be just as easily—and perhaps more appropriately—be translated as "blood of another." Given such ambiguity and alternate pronoun substitution, verse 4 might read quite differently, even portraying a hunter-prey relationship.

---

158 Genesis 1:29-30, Genesis 9:3, Leviticus 11, Deuteronomy 14

159 The masculine pronoun also suggests preferential use of male animals for food or sacrifice, e.g., 1 Chronicles 29:21 and Malachi 1:14. Also, mothers are forbidden to be used as food, e.g., Deuteronomy 22:6-7. Mothers might also be understood to have the "blood of another" in them (as with human babies, cattle embryo blood types are determined paternally, thus it differs from the mother's blood). http://www. ilri.cgiar.org/InfoServ/Webpub/fulldocs/X5443E/X5443E19.HTM

Only the flesh with *another's blood in its soul* do not eat.
(Gen. 9: 4 AHT)[160]

Instead of seeing this Genesis 9:4 text as yet another distinction between kosher and unkosher animals, Jews and Christians alike fail to see the false dichotomy, i.e., "either-or" commitments made in pronoun association. Thus, they typically attribute this text exclusively to the practice of draining the blood from animals post-slaughter.[161]

Lifeblood and Bloody Meat

While most translations assume that Genesis 9:4 pronouns are referring to one and the same animal, to assume that the text is only referring to post-slaughter blood drainage is perhaps presumptuous. Nevertheless, the favoring of the blood draining interpretation is apparent in the NIV translation as cited on page 115, as a superfluous "still" term was interjected in order to further allude to blood draining processes, even though the original Hebrew not does include words to imply "still" or "remaining." However, it is also interesting that in this post-flood blessing context, no particular butchering, hanging, or salting procedures are prescribed for the sake of blood draining or evacuation, as is the case of other texts prohibiting blood consumption.[162] Furthermore, it is also worth considering that any such blood removal processes are incapable of removing every last drop of blood from an animal, making absolute and literal blood evacuation fulfillment a difficult feat and the common pronoun interpretation more suspect.

---

160 Author's translation

161 Jewish Noahide laws to prohibit the consumption of blood or limbs from living animals are inferred from this verse, and Christians often associate it with Acts 15, which contains James's prohibition to "abstain from blood."

162 Post-slaughter blood draining methods in the written Torah are not defined in conjunction with any other texts that prohibit blood consumption outright, such as Leviticus 7:26, 17:10-14, 19:26, Deuteronomy 12:16-24, and 15:23; although Leviticus 17:13 prescribes that blood that is poured out is to be covered with earth.

While there is indeed biblical and scientific[163] merit to the traditional blood draining interpretation, it is also likely that post-slaughter blood evacuation is not the greater intention of the message encapsulated within the original Genesis 9:4 Hebrew text. In fact, as the verses are paired together with a proper translation of the previous verse, it becomes even clearer that Noah wasn't given "everything moving" to eat. To the contrary, the animals created for man were given for food *because* they ate green herbs and ate no blood.

> Everything moving which lives for you, it will be for food *according to* the green herbs; I gave to you every such thing. Only the flesh with *another's blood in its soul* do not eat. (Gen. 9:3–4 AHT)[164]

While there is good reason to recognize both the blood draining and the "another's blood" interpretations in Genesis 9:4 as concurrently legitimate, as suggested by the two differing "ו" (vav) pronoun interpretations, it also stands to reason that the "blood of another" interpretation is consistent with the differing anatomical traits and dietary instincts of clean and unclean animals vaguely distinguished within the original Genesis creation account. Likewise, unclean animals with traits as described in Leviticus 11 are those that eat other animals or whose carcasses have short digestive tracts, which are also capable of rapidly processing the flesh and blood of their prey—unlike those feeding exclusively on greens and plant-based foods, which are equipped with long digestive tracts to process grasses and other forms of fibrous vegetation.

As a carnivore binges on another animal or decomposing carcass, it is possible that the blood of the victim directly shunts into the bloodstream of the predator. Whether the blood of the prey is digested in the stomach or passes into the bloodstream of the predator, either way it is inevitable that the blood of the prey enters into the unclean

---

163 Failure to promptly drain blood from a slaughtered animal results in meat spoilage.
164 Author's translation

animal. Thus, it is reasonable to conclude that unclean animals can be described as animals that "have the 'lifeblood' (of another animal) in them," especially as many unclean animals are hematophagous by nature, feeding on the blood of their prey—some of them even doing so exclusively.

After blessing humanity as the apex of creation in Eden—and after flood re-creation—God gave them food. In the beginning, God made some clean animals "living for" people to eat, which are those that ate green herbs. He also made unclean animals to clean up the road kill left behind by any other animals, including the "life-blood," the guts, and everything else, which was not to be eaten by man.[165] These principles held true in the time of Adam, Noah, and Moses, just as they remain true today.

Green is Clean, Red is Dead, and White may be Right

Although Noah had ample foreknowledge, he was nevertheless reminded after the flood that as a general guideline, the "green meat" (grazing vegetarian diet) animal varieties were clean and acceptable to eat;[166] the "red meat" (carnivorous diet) animals were unclean and forbidden to eat. It's a simple system: green is clean and red is dead. Like traffic lights, green is "go," and red is "no go." Green eggs are fine to eat, but green ham must be rejected as a work of fiction—not even remotely suitable for a child's entertainment. The earth's ecosystems are dependent on these relationships; cycles of life cannot be completed without both animal types. There is no reason to invoke miracles and infer changes to animal anatomy or physiology in pre-flood times or while the animals remained in the ark. Likewise, there is no evidence, be it derived from Scriptural, scientific, or secular sources, to suggest any sort of animal transition at the time of the flood. Unclean animals are designed—from the very beginning—to eat clean animals with the

---

165 Exodus 22:31

166 Grazing animals such as horses do not fit kosher criterion per Leviticus 11, and they also eat fruit, which is contrary to Genesis 1 standards.

unique exception of fish, which are for good reasons not described in either the Adamic or Noahic blessing.

As far as kosher animal types are concerned, fish fit into a special category, as they are constantly immersed in water and not restricted to vegetarian diets, unlike their clean green-eating, air-breathing counterparts. Like their kosher air-breathing, green-eating counterparts, finned-and-scaled clean fish varieties do not dine on decomposing matter, even though many of them do regularly dine on unclean aquatic species. While unclean aquatic creatures, such as shellfish, sharks, eels, catfish, and other fish types without scales and fins, are generally willing to scavenge on decomposing creatures, their flesh is white and not laden with blood. Likewise, the flesh or meat of the clean fish is not full of blood. Thus, meat derived from clean fish cannot be described as fish with the "lifeblood still in it," or as flesh with another's blood in its soul. In other words, as far as fish are concerned, "white is all right" for human food, provided there are fins and scales surrounding the white meat.

Given this contrast between aquatic and air breathing creatures, it is interesting that Peter's vision coincided with distinctions in food blessings to Adam and Noah. While Peter's vision included quadrupeds, birds, and crawling things, he makes no mention of fish in his visions, even though he was a fisherman by vocation.[167] Thus it is reasonable to assert that all of the three food-related blessings where food types are qualified—including Adam's, Noah's, and Peter's—are equally misinterpreted and abused to undermine a kosher worldview!

Wild and Domestic – According to their Kinds

In addition to describing the four principal animal types based on their domains, the Genesis account makes subtle allusion to clean and unclean "kinds." Although many readers may legitimately interpret animal "kinds" as species variation within animal kingdoms, the text may certainly also refer to "clean and unclean" when it speaks of animals

---

167 Acts 10

created according to their "kinds." As a help to Adam, Noah, and all later generations, God created two animal kinds with distinct natural traits such that casual observers of nature might distinguish between them and make use of their observations.

Inherently practical to domesticate, the clean and edible kinds of non-aquatic animals may be described as:

✓ Communal (social to each other, inclined to herd)
✓ Defensive (good peripheral vision for self-preservation)
✓ Nurturing (caring for and never eating their young)
✓ Passive or gentle (not aggressive unless threatened)
✓ Unintelligent (easy to corral, feed, shear, and slaughter)
✓ Slow (usually easy to catch and domesticate)
✓ Grazing (feeding exclusively on grass or vegetation)
✓ Hygienic (usually in contact with fresh food and generating relatively nontoxic wastes; not disease-hosting)
✓ Non-hematophagous (no appetite for blood)

Though the English term *livestock* may lack direct biblical correlation or equivalence to any Hebrew word, the term has great value in describing clean animals suitable for domestication. Clean animals can serve as an excellent living store of nutrition and can survive on dry grass during winter or drought.

In contrast, unclean animals have radically different demeanors. Most unclean kinds may be described as:

✓ Independent (lone, but possibly joining hunting packs)
✓ Offensive (fangs, claws, poison, vision for hunting)
✓ Nomadic (migrating for prey, inclined to abandon young)
✓ Hostile or aggressive (posing lethal threats to people)
✓ Cunning (inclined to study and stalk prey)
✓ Fast (often difficult to catch and domesticate)
✓ Scavenging (may eat rotting flesh; may be cannibalistic)
✓ Unhygienic (often in contact with meat in states of decomposition, generating parasite-laden toxic wastes)

✓ Hematophagous (consuming blood)

Even though the English term *wild* may lack perfect correlation with Hebrew animal terms in the Bible, the word does nevertheless describe most unclean animals. Whereas clean animals serve as excellent livestock, unclean animals are instrumental in keeping undomesticated clean animal herds within healthy natural limits, even cleansing the earth of the remains of the dead. Obviously, each animal kind is created according to its purpose, just as each animal kind is given the demeanor to match. Noah surely understood this before the storm brewed or the rain fell, just as Adam did as he named the animals in the beginning.

Shepherding Flocks outside of Eden

To assert that ancient knowledge of clean and unclean animals in the pre-flood world and other dining stipulations was inferior, or completely lost forever in the sands of time—or in the waters of the flood—is fishy doctrine as farfetched as it is unbelievable. In the time between Noah and Moses, there is no reason to believe that Abraham, Isaac, and Jacob were deprived of such ancient foreknowledge; they were not known for herding pigs and eating pork. To the contrary, the knowledge of these blessings was, at a minimum, carried orally from the time of Adam to Noah's day, much as information would later be relayed from Noah to Abraham. [168] In fact, it is evident that Cain and Abel lived in accordance with the very same dining blessings given to their father Adam.

Little is recorded in Genesis about Abel, Adam's son, the second born in the human race. Yet from the little that is written, it is only

---

168 Per Genesis 9:28–29, 11:10–26, it is probable that Abraham knew Noah, given the Genesis lineages, life spans, and timelines presented. Jasher 12:63 and Jasher 12:69 imply interaction. See Joshua 10:13, 2 Samuel 1:18, and 2 Timothy 3:8 for Jasher references.

prudent to conclude that Abel consumed kosher animals.[169] The Genesis account reads,

> But Abel brought fat portions from some of the firstborn of his flock. The Lord looked with favor on Abel and his offering. (Gen. 4:4)

This text, however minuscule and trivial it may appear, reveals interesting facts directly pertaining to the timeless kosher argument. From this text, it is easy to deduce that:

✓ Abel was a shepherd.
✓ Abel offered firstborn animals.
✓ Abel retained animals beyond what he offered.
✓ Abel offered fattened portions.
✓ Abel pleased God by his actions.

These few isolated facts pave the road to several questions and discussions, all of which lend credence to interpretations that support the notion of everlasting human kosher omnivore diets.

Abel's Leftover Animals

A simple proof contrary to the Genesis "first family" vegan or vegetarian view is one of animal surplus. The first question raised by Genesis 4:4 might be, aside from the portion offered in sacrifice, what did Abel do with the surplus animals in his flock? If Abel was sacrificing only the fattened firstborn of his flock, what did he do with the rest of the animals?

Those promoting a vegetarian worldview and opposing the ancient use of surplus animals for kosher culinary purposes may reason that Abel kept his surplus herds exclusively for clothing. But this argument

---

169 Aside from Genesis allusions cited herein, Jasher 1:19–20 alludes to Cain's use of Abel's animals for human food purposes.

begs another question: why wouldn't Abel grow cotton or hemp to make linen garments instead of using animal-based materials, such as wool or leather?

Most scholars seem to share the opinion that before the flood, the earth's climate was temperate.[170] If this is the case, the suitability of Abel's vocation relative to the environment must be considered. If he kept flocks exclusively for making sacrifices and clothing, did he use the animals for leather or only for wool? A clothing-shepherd explanation of Abel does not consider that there are valid substitute plant-based materials, such as cotton or linen, which are arguably more suitable for wearing in temperate environments. But this begs another more important question: what of Adam and Eve's garments relative to Abel's vocation?

Eden's Tannery and Textiles

Much like Cain made an unacceptable fruit-based offering, so too did Adam and Eve try using plant-based garments—leaves from a fig tree—to cover their naked bodies. For whatever reason, God deemed the fig leaves insufficient; and in response, he gave Adam and Eve leather garments to wear.[171] The animal type used by God is not identified, but it is clear from the Genesis account, however curious it may be, that God expected Adam and Eve to wear leather. It may be extreme to propose that Adam, Eve, and their offspring were forbidden to wear fabric derived from plants, like cotton or linen, but clearly, the use of animals for clothing materials, whether leather or wool, is not without divine precedent. God would not break his own "no killing animals for utilitarian purposes" rule, as inferred and promoted by vegans dedicated to dogmatic religious persuasions, to clothe Adam and Eve while expecting Adam's children to do otherwise.

Furthermore, the clothing-shepherd explanation fails to address the question of quantity, need, and surplus of Abel's flock. After all, how

---

170 A mild earth climate might be inferred from Genesis 1:7 or 2:6.
171 Genesis 3:7, 21

much leather or wool could Abel possibly use to clothe himself and his family? Granted, Adam and Eve may have needed little clothing, if the cartoons that show them in skimpy fig-leaf costumes are correct, even though there is reason to believe they were wearing modest animal hides for the majority of their lives. As for Abel, regardless of the size of the loincloths he made, how large could his wardrobe possibly have been? Would he have needed multitudes of flocks to clothe himself, given the climate? Did Abel curtail the size of the flock to meet his needs as a textile maker, tailor, or leather smith?

Finally, the question of timing must be considered. As for the surplus animals that Abel withheld from sacrifice and may have used for clothing, did he slaughter them or wait for them to die of natural causes before harvesting the leather? And if he slaughtered them for the sake of leather, did Abel—supposedly born as a pre-flood vegetarian—leave the meat to rot in the field, or was he obligated instead to feed it to some unclean wild animal that he had dominion over, which supposedly was created as vegan also? Even if Abel were using leather hides for tent construction while his brother Cain was building a brick-and-mortar city, he eventually would have exhausted his need for leather canvas, and his flock, if he was indeed a strict vegan.

Abel's Fattened Flock

While it may be idealistic and heartwarming for some people to entertain vegetarian-clothing-shepherd views of Abel and the rest of ancient humanity, only the explanation that ancient humanity were kosher omnivores is compatible with the Genesis 4:4 text. After all, the Scriptures say that Abel offered the "fat portions" of his flock. As described in other texts, the fat portions were those most desired for eating and were reserved for divine allotment or special celebration. Conversely, the fattened animals are not revered anywhere in the text for being exceptional milk, wool, or leather producers. This view of the fattened calf being favorable for food is consistent with numerous portions of Moses' Torah and the Psalms, just as it is with gospel accounts.[172] Thus, to suggest that Abel was not eating kosher meats—from the beginning—is every bit as ridiculous as suggesting that he was a hobby farmer who kept his surplus sheep for pets and occasional religious or recreational sacrifice. Suggesting such implies that there was nothing special about the fattened animals Abel offered.

Finally, if Adam and subsequent ancient generations were not permitted or blessed to use animals for food until after the flood, but only green-seed plant life, why would God be pleased with Abel, given that he was working as a shepherd? To suggest that early humanity ate nothing more than apples after being ejected from Eden is hardly valid. Such a vegan-man view is unacceptable and even akin to advocating Cain's unacceptable fruit sacrifice; it discounts Abel's honest shepherding vocation, his superior offering, and God's favor toward him.

Shiny Rotten Apples of Eden

Children and adults of all ages are equally perplexed by the Adam and Eve "forbidden fruit" account. From the standpoint of logic or human intuition, the injustice isn't obvious or apparent—it's almost foreign to the imagination. It incites curiosity and leaves people flustered. What was it about that fruit? Why was it forbidden? Was the fruit poisoned? Was it somehow evil? Why didn't God issue "more important" commands to Adam and Eve like "don't steal" or "don't murder"? At one time or another, almost everyone has wondered why the fruit wasn't kosher, or why it was forbidden. Even standing from today's vantage point with 20/20 hindsight, people reluctantly accept the fact that eating the forbidden fruit caused death.

Believers today are given the grace by which to make a different choice; they can respond to the mysterious kosher commands in reverent humility or with rebellious hostility.

As for the fruit of Eden, there was a particular tree in the middle of the garden that was clearly not kosher to eat at any time, despite the earlier Genesis endorsement of all seeded fruits for human consumption.

---

172 Leviticus 3:16, Psalm 66:15, Luke 15

Even before the fall, God disqualified some particular fruits as food, deeming them to be unkosher.

> And the Lord God commanded the man, "You are free to eat from any tree in the garden; but you must not eat from the tree of the knowledge of good and evil, for when you eat of it you will surely die." (Gen. 2:16–17)

As the story goes, the man took no action to compel the woman to refrain from eating the fruit. The Genesis text reveals,

> When the woman saw that the fruit of the tree was good for food and pleasing to the eye, and also desirable for gaining wisdom, she took some and ate it. (Gen. 3:6)

As for color or type, nobody knows what the forbidden fruit looked like. Artists commonly portray it, for whatever reason, as an apple, perhaps because *apple* begins with the first letter of the English alphabet and is synonymous with the remedial learning of early Genesis, which describes things that were "in the beginning." Usually depicted as red in color and lush in appearance, the apple is striking, universally recognized, and unlike any other fruit.

Yet perhaps the apple is portrayed as the forbidden fruit for an even deeper reason—its deceptive potential. Behind that shiny skin, the fruit's flesh is assumed to be crisp, juicy, and sweet. Still, when it comes to eating apples, everyone has been duped by false appearances. At times, even though they look great on the outside, apples are soft, grainy, or sour, making them suitable only for applesauce, apple cider vinegar, or animal food. Worse yet, a healthy-looking apple can serve as food and lodging for a worm or other parasite. Such is the case with dispensational teaching. After all, much dispensational teaching looks great on the surface, but in the end, the flesh of such fruit is unclean and worm-infested to the very core.

Deceiving the Woman

Regardless of the type of fruit growing on Eden's forbidden tree, a deceitful appearance is cited as one of the two factors that contributed to Eve's deception, the other being the pursuit of wisdom apart from God's commandments. Eve was tricked into thinking that 'food' was in the eye of the beholder. Rather than deferring to her husband to clarify the divine revelation, she embarked on an independent path of lawlessness and moral relativism, contrary to what she knew was right, in hopes of liberating and elevating herself. Because it looked like 'food' to her, Eve ate the fruit. No doubt it was appealing, and she might have even enjoyed the taste. Nevertheless, the forbidden fruit should never have been considered 'food.'

Of course, Adam's participation in Eve's deception must be kept in proper perspective; for it was Adam that received the first "false fruit" warning directly from God. Such a privilege would not only make Adam responsible for Eve's instruction, but also accountable for Eve's actions - especially given Adam's presence during Eve's seduction. For good reason, this Garden of Eden account might also serve as a lasting example of bad church/clergy relationships, with Adam's apathetic actions compared to those of a passive and complacent clergy. Obviously, when a "husband" of any sort fails to teach and live by God's commandments, "the bride" will suffer the same fate as did Eve, who was left uncorrected and ungrounded in the truth of God's word, which made her especially vulnerable to evil's false fruits and tempting promises.

Whether leader or follower, those consenting to dispensational dining views of various Scripture narratives have, in effect, been deceived, and have eaten forbidden, unclean, and unkosher 'food' as Adam and Eve did. Tricked by crafty dispensational serpents and ignorant shepherds, congregants have been enticed to disregard the list of forbidden foods in Leviticus 11— in the same way that Eve was fooled into eating the forbidden fruit of Genesis chapters 2 and 3—by half-truths and out-of-context citations. Rather than asking, "Did God really say, 'You must not eat from any tree in the garden'?" dispensational theologians are now applying different tactics. They tamper with New Testament texts, asserting, "Didn't Jesus declare all foods clean? Didn't God say that Peter should get up and kill and eat everything? Didn't James say that only strangled animals were to be avoided as food? Didn't Paul say that all foods are clean?"

Sober Priests and Bible Food

While people usually associate kosher commandments with Moses, the responsibility of kosher teaching and oversight actually went to Moses' brother Aaron and his sons, who were appointed by God to serve as priests. Although Aaron and Moses received the divine dietary regulations concurrently,[173] it is probable that Aaron was more likely to take them to heart than was Moses. Unfortunately for Aaron, he would hear these commandments not long after witnessing divine judgment fall on two sons who failed to properly perform their duties.[174] To say the least, this sobering event would leave both the circumstances and the commandments strongly imprinted in his mind.

Expecting priests to minister with discernment and their full mental faculties, the LORD first prescribed the unique priestly expectations to Aaron and his family, providing a priestly charter statement.

> You and your sons are not to drink wine or other fermented drink whenever you go into the Tent of Meeting, or you will die. This is a lasting ordinance for the generations to come. You must distinguish between the holy and the common, between the unclean and the clean, and you must teach the Israelites all the decrees the Lord has given them through Moses. (Lev. 10:9–11)

---

173 Leviticus 11:1

174 Sequential chronology is assumed in the Leviticus 10 account. Some believe that Aaron's sons were ministering in an impaired state per Leviticus 10:9; others suggest they were sober per Deuteronomy 29:6.

The first half of the vocational charter that was assigned to Aaron and his sons as priests was to teach the Israelites to distinguish between the unclean and the clean. The remaining half of the charter was dedicated to teaching other commandments. Even though there are no sons of Aaron actively presiding over the office of the priesthood today, surely the emphasis and scope of the priestly charter must not be disregarded as irrelevant. Citing offensive and dysfunctional religious authorities more than two thousand years ago, Ezekiel spoke in the first person and on behalf of God himself, saying,

> Her priests do violence to my law and profane my holy things; they do not distinguish between the holy and the common; they teach that there is no difference between the unclean and the clean. (Ezek. 22:26)

Because the law of Moses remains in effect and because no New Testament figure came to overturn that law,[175] it stands to reason that Aaron's charter for ministers and Ezekiel's prophetic indictment of substandard ministry remain relevant to this day. Ministers of modern times—who are not priests—might take note of Ezekiel's rebuke and Aaron's charter; anyone professing to teach the word of God will ultimately be critiqued on their ability to uphold the charter of distinguishing between the clean and the unclean, while instructing their audiences to do the same. In accordance with these texts, apostate ministers who are committed to teaching contrary to Moses' law must be called to account. After all, Jesus could never be revered as a "priest on the order of Melchizedek"[176] or as the "prophet likened unto Moses"[177] if he could not do something as simple and prudent as distinguish between the clean and the unclean, as Aaron and Moses did. Moreover, according to gospel texts, those claiming to teach and follow in Jesus' footsteps while eating unclean foods and teaching that there is no

---

175 Matthew 5:17
176 Hebrews 5:6
177 Deuteronomy 18:15–18

difference between the clean and the unclean will be called least in the kingdom of heaven.[178]

Rules and Reasons for Children

Perhaps this kosher message is most difficult for clergy and congregants to accept because unimpeded and unprecedented gluttony has become the norm in Western civilization and churches; people cannot fathom that God would impose or maintain any dietary restrictions. Adam and Eve's single failure didn't make the fruit acceptable to later generations, nor did Jesus' crucifixion remove forbidden food from the planet. A response of rebellion to such plain and simple truths is nothing less than childish. Theologians who say something like, "Go ahead; put anything in your mouth!" must be flagged for endorsing suspicious and reckless behavior; such clergy have obviously failed to learn and accept the most rudimentary Genesis lesson of Adam and Eve. Such theologians are doing exactly what the serpent did.

Children are rightly conditioned and corrected in response to a dangerous behavior that starts even before they learn to speak. Even prior to learning how to crawl, children are told time and time again, "Don't put that thing in your mouth!" Of course, parents understand what children do not—that food is not defined by the mouth's mere ability to receive it, and that sampling things with no guidelines or discretion can be downright deadly. Any parent knows that something does not automatically become food just because it can be tasted, chewed, swallowed, or digested.

Fortunately for young children, parents are loving, patient, and not quickly angered when they experiment without comprehension, putting nonfood or dangerous items into their mouths. Despite repetition of dangerous behavior, children receive unconditional forgiveness because of their ignorance or undeveloped powers of comprehension.

However, ignorance is no excuse in the case of an older child, who can comprehend, or an adult, who should know better. Ignorance is

---

178 Matthew 5:19

forgivable, but rebellion against good laws established by a good God is just plain stupidity. While the prophet Hosea said, "My people perish for the lack of knowledge,"[179] the prophet Samuel likened rebellion to witchcraft.[180] Ignorance is one path to destruction, but it is probably safe to say that rebellion is a faster route to much greater devastation.

Only after being expelled from the Garden of Eden would Adam and Eve consent to view food from the proper divine perspective. Surely for centuries following their ejection from Eden, they would stop and think twice before putting something into their mouths. And they wouldn't pay much attention to snake oil salesmen pushing bad theology and asking, "Did God really say that?" Instead, they would listen to their Father, who said in the beginning, "Don't eat that because I said so!"and even, "Don't eat that because it will kill you!"

---

179 Hosea 4:6
180 1 Samuel 15:23

Chapter 4 Notes

Chapter 4 Notes

5

Translations for Every Appetite

Do not add to what I command you and do not subtract from it, but keep the commands of the LORD your God that I give you.

—Deut. 4:2

Every word of God is flawless; he is a shield to those who take refuge in him. Do not add to his words, or he will rebuke you and prove you a liar.

—Prov. 30:5-6

I warn everyone who hears the words of the prophecy of this book: If anyone adds anything to them, God will add to him the plagues described in this book. And if anyone takes words away from this book of prophecy, God will take away from him his share in the tree of life and in the holy city, which are described in this book.

—Rev. 22:18-19

Afte examining essential food-related Scriptures in their original languages and greater contexts, it becomes apparent that many Bible texts have been interpreted and translated incorrectly – with a strong dispensational and unkosher bias. Furthermore, it is evident that the relationship between Bible misinterpretation and mistranslation is a vicious circle, where misinterpretation prompts mistranslation, which in turn only feeds more misinterpretation.

Translation Errors—Origins and Implications

For obvious reasons, the quality of a Bible translation is always limited by the quality of a Bible interpretation; but conversely, the validity of a Bible interpretation might be independent of a Bible translation. In other words, things such as human inference, preconceived notions, and finite knowledge can all influence the interpretation of Bible texts, potentially compromising the meaning irrespective of manuscript vintage or language. For example, the understanding of contexts, ancient cultures, history, geography, and even science might all contribute to the meaning of a chapter, verse, or a given word. Consequently, it is to be expected that errors in interpretation might either precede or succeed Bible translation errors.

However, apart from the factors potentially contributing to misinterpretation as described above, translation errors may also stem from an imperfect understanding of ancient languages. In fact, translators repeatedly confess to limited knowledge of the ancient languages, even candidly admitting uncertainty within the footnotes of English Bibles. These cases, however, fail to capture the cases where the translator—even with the best of intentions—had the wrong conviction from the beginning. Moreover, it is also safe to say that no translator will have a perfect understanding of the original and divinely inspired messages; as a result, the accuracy of all Bible translations is further compromised.

Needless to say, even the most diligent English Bible readers can easily fall victim to errors in translation, especially if they are fully dependent on a single Bible translation. As readers try to interpret the English texts through the eyes of translators, they are left vulnerable to assumptions and conjecture far more than they may realize. In effect, English readers are ultimately forced to try to overcome problems of ignorance by ingesting imperfect information as imparted into their Bible translations—not knowing where or to what extent their study might be prejudiced by a translator's initial assumptions or influenced by a lack of knowledge. Without divine intervention or diligent examination, translation errors are hard for an English-only reader to identify; they are almost certain to balloon into colossal zeppelins of misinterpretation. Such is the case with translations and interpretations related to dispensational dining doctrines.

Tables of Interpretation

To help illustrate how presumptive dispensational misinterpretations have produced mistranslations, which in turn have contributed to even greater misinterpretations, Table 5 below includes a summary of points discussed in earlier chapters, contrasting true forms (+) of kosher Christianity against false (-) dispensational food related doctrines. Although Table 5 does not differentiate between errors of interpretation and errors of translation, the summary of accounts below will nevertheless help illustrate how just a few minor and unkosher mistranslations, like those of Genesis 1 and Mark 7, can influence the interpretation and thought progression throughout the entire Bible narrative.

TABLE 3 –
KOSHER CHRISTIANITY VS
DISPENSATIONAL CHRISTIANITY

Kosher Christianity	Text	Dispensational Christianity
+ God defines only human food + Man blessed with omnivore diet + Man's diet includes herbivores	Adam Gen. 1	- God defined foods for all animals - Man created as vegan - God creates only vegan animals
+ Abel keeps clean animals to eat + Cain ate of Abel's animal flock + Abel raises animals for leather + Abel eats dairy products	Abel Gen. 4	- All people were vegan until Noah - Abel's animals only for sacrifice - Shepherding is only for wool - Abel eats but fruits & vegetables
+ Seven clean animal pairs on Ark + Noah's blessing same as Adam's + Herbivores remain food for man + Blood carnivores banned as food	Noah Gen. 7 Gen. 9	- Single pairs of all Ark animals - Noah received a new blessing - Noah's family first to eat animals - Man given any animal to eat
+ God details eternal food laws + Israel's laws good for all nations	Moses Lev. 11	- New temporary food laws given - Kosher laws given to Jews only
+ Daniel avoided defiled meat + Daniel avoided unclean meat + Daniel avoided absinthe wine	Daniel Dan. 1	- Vegan diets are superior - Daniel avoided "royal" foods - All alcohol is forbidden
+ Jesus did not cleanse foods + Jesus rejected elder's customs + Jesus spoke about digestion + Improper washing is insufficient + Pharisees ignored Moses' law + Bodily fluids are still unclean + Evil is not from dirty food + Evil is not from unwashed hands	Jesus Mk. 7 Mat.15	- Jesus declared all food clean - Jesus repealed Moses' law - Jesus called everything edible - Washing is no longer relevant - Christians can ignore Moses' law - Uncleanness is only spiritual - Eating bad food is harmless - Eating forbidden food is not evil

Kosher Christianity	Text	Dispensational Christianity
+ Animal vision is about bigotry + Peter saw clean/unclean animals + Peter calls clean animals "defiled" + Peter rejects clean animals + Peter never ate unclean foods + Peter's sees own bigotry in vision + Peter repents of his own bigotry	Peter Acts 10	- Animal vision redefines food - Peter saw only unclean animals - God calls unclean animals clean - Peter's rejection is baseless - Peter disobeyed Jesus (Mark 7) - Peter sees all animals are food - Peter eats all unclean animals
+ Idolatry can defile people + Blood ban includes unclean meat + Gentiles directed to Moses' law + Leviticus given as starting point + Spirit acts without man's counsel	James Acts 15	- Idols can defile food - Only drinking blood forbidden - Gentiles relieved of Moses' law - Only 4 laws retained for Gentiles - Spirit treated as equal member
+ Food defined in Gen. 1 & Lev. 11 + Unclean things can defile food + Clean food can't defile itself + Man should reject defiled food + Veganism is not biblical doctrine	Paul Rom. 14	- Food is defined by dictionary - Unclean food is imaginary - Defiled food is imaginary - Man should receive all as food - Belief in Jesus cleans any food
+ Not everything edible is "food" + Idols can't defile food anywhere + People are defiled by idol worship	Paul 1 Cor 8	- Eat anything served to you - Eat anything from meat market - Food can be defiled by idols
+ Taste anything clean and kosher + Man made rules are self-affliction + Obeying Moses' law pleases God + Dogma is based on human ideas + Dogma was "nailed to the cross" + Moses' law to remain forever + Unclean food is harsh upon body	Paul Col 2	- Taste anything whatsoever - Moses' law is self-affliction - Moses' law is false humility - Moses' law is man-made dogma - Moses' law was crucified - Moses' law is destined to perish - Food laws cause bodily hardship
+ Kosher things are food + Kosher food not to be forbidden + Heretics forbid kosher food	Paul 1 Tim 4	- All things are food - Kosher restrictions are demonic - Heretics forbid unclean food

Although food-related comments in 1 Timothy 4 and Colossians 2 were not addressed in prior chapters, the contrasting kosher and dispensational views of these passages are briefly contrasted in the table above, where the same principles apply to interpretation as in earlier New Testament texts.

Translation Dispensations

As demonstrated in the table above, several minor misinterpretations and mistranslations have a permeating impact on the Bible's overall message. The kosher views are consistent with a god that says, "I change not"; the dispensational views leave mankind befuddled with respect to standards of morality and food. Generations holding unkosher views, not being anchored in absolute distinctions between right and wrong, are forced to wrestle with varied dining instructions and dispensations, taking a host of confused people from extreme vegan to unlimited smorgasbord diets.

Figure 2 below illustrates and compares the kosher views to the dispensations assumed by proponents of unkosher views, in order to demonstrate the unreliability of dispensational dining doctrines. Fickle dispensational tendencies are made evident in many translations and traditional interpretations.

FIGURE 2 – PROPOSED DIETARY DISPENSATIONS

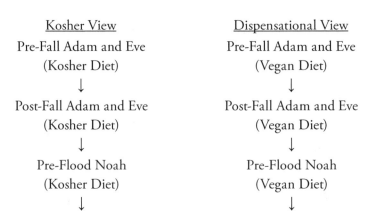

Kosher View	Dispensational View
Pre-Fall Adam and Eve	Pre-Fall Adam and Eve
(Kosher Diet)	(Vegan Diet)
↓	↓
Post-Fall Adam and Eve	Post-Fall Adam and Eve
(Kosher Diet)	(Vegan Diet)
↓	↓
Pre-Flood Noah	Pre-Flood Noah
(Kosher Diet)	(Vegan Diet)
↓	↓

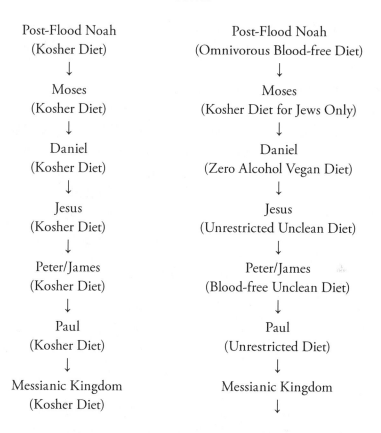

Post-Flood Noah (Kosher Diet) ↓	Post-Flood Noah (Omnivorous Blood-free Diet) ↓
Moses (Kosher Diet) ↓	Moses (Kosher Diet for Jews Only) ↓
Daniel (Kosher Diet) ↓	Daniel (Zero Alcohol Vegan Diet) ↓
Jesus (Kosher Diet) ↓	Jesus (Unrestricted Unclean Diet) ↓
Peter/James (Kosher Diet) ↓	Peter/James (Blood-free Unclean Diet) ↓
Paul (Kosher Diet) ↓	Paul (Unrestricted Diet) ↓
Messianic Kingdom (Kosher Diet)	Messianic Kingdom ↓

As the dispensational confusion mounts throughout the Bible narrative, it becomes clear that even the early Genesis mistranslations and misinterpretations presented herein cannot be dismissed as merely theoretical, historical, or even trivial in nature.

It is ultimately the interpretations and the translations of New Testament texts that are likely to have the greatest bearing on a Christian's everyday life. After all, when Christians are presented with Jesus' testimony and identity, they are likely to accept his words as authoritative—some even believing his words were recorded to supersede other Bible texts. Thus, Christians look to New Testament texts for moral reasoning and direction, believing that Jesus' words are of greater significance than—and sometimes even contrary to—other Bible texts.

Regrettably, people forget that English was not Jesus' native tongue, not realizing that what they believe to be Jesus' words are, in fact, mere English translations of the original New Testament texts. From these bad English renderings, Christians presume that Jesus granted them permission to renounce all food laws, which were otherwise in effect up until his incarnation, crucifixion, or ascension. As a result, mistranslations of Mark 7 have become more than a wayward point of origin; they have become the broken compass by which all Bible food doctrines are oriented. These mistranslations may be likened to an offset rudder that has been used to set the course of titanic dining doctrines whereby the entire crew arrives at the wrong destination, along with an unclean breakfast menu.

Tables of Translation

Given the New International Version's growing popularity and influence within Christian theology today, it was fitting to exhibit the translation's dispensational bias present in Mark 7 as well as in the other verses. However, *EAT LIKE JESUS* should by no means be construed as a malicious assault on one particular Bible translation.[181] After all, the dispensational theology that debases the NIV can hardly be attributed to a small multidenominational translation committee deliberating on a handful of verses. In fact, many of the NIV's dispensational slants are anything but original, as dispensational dogma and anti-kosher worldviews have been prevalent in Christianity and Bible versions for generations prior to the NIV's inception.

---

181 Widespread NIV usage demonstrates Christendom's extensive conformance to dispensational doctrines. Composed by dozens of theologians from dozens of denominations and institutions, the NIV is credited as being accepted by more denominations than any other translation. As the world's best selling Bible, NIV sales account for over one-third of Bible sales worldwide, having sold over 400 million copies since publication in 1978. Thus, the NIV is probably the most representative of Christian thinking, as well as the greatest influence upon Christian teaching and doctrine.
http://www.biblica.com/niv/translators/
http://www.amazon.com/Zondervan-NIV-Study-Bible/dp/0310929555
http://www.nbcnews.com/id/32644719/ns/us_news-faith/#.USqfKDCOB_c
http://books.google.com/books/about/Holy_Bible_NIV.html?id=JjGiGOYJLoYC

But what about these other English Bible translations? How do they interpret Jesus' precedent-setting Mark 7 dining revelations? Do they also propose that "Jesus declared all foods clean"? Do they suggest that every kind of animal was to be considered "clean" food? Do they assert that food can no longer be made dirty if handled in an unhygienic fashion? Do they describe the caustic purification caused by the human digestion process—whereby foods are "cleansed" and "purged" as they pass through and are expelled from the body?

In response to these questions, English renderings of Mark 7:19 from over forty of the most popular and respected Bible translations[182] have been included in tables below for purposes of comparison and consideration. Apart from obvious dispensational biases and overtones, it would appear that differences in translation are defined by the following variances:

- ✓ Quotation mark placement – Based on Greek text punctuation, different translations interpret differing endpoints of Jesus' words in verse 19.
- ✓ Commentary – Based on Greek text punctuation and endpoints of Jesus' words, some translations assume that concluding words are gospel writers' commentary.
- ✓ Interjection / substitution – Most translations employ words dissimilar from the original Greek text to help substantiate views on punctuation and commentary.

Given such variation, popular English Bible translations have been grouped into two different sets of tables below—one that assumes the entirety of the Mark 7:19 Greek text (see page 18 of chapter 1 for interlinear presentation) should be interpreted as Jesus' words without commentary (Table 4), and the other (Table 5) that assumes the four concluding Greek words of Mark 7:19 are to be rendered as gospel author commentary on Jesus' preceding statement.

---

182 Numbers are added to Table 4 and Table 5 to identify nine of the top ten bestselling English Bibles according to Association for Christian Retail statistics, http://www.cbaonline.org/nm/documents/bsls/bible_translations.pdf

TABLE 4—
MARK 7:19 TRANSLATED AS
JESUS' WORDS ONLY

Translation	Mark 7:19 Interpretation
1587 Geneva Bible	Because it entreth not into his heart, but into the belly, and goeth out into the draught which is the purging of all meates?
1611 King James [#2]	Because it entreth not into his heart, but into the belly, and goeth out into the draught, purging all meats?
Modern King James	Because it does not enter into his heart, but into the belly, and goes out into the waste-bowl, purifying all food?
New King James [#4]	because it does not enter his heart but his stomach, and is eliminated, thus purifying all foods?"[a] NKJV footnote: a. Mark 7:19 NU-Text ends quotation with eliminated, setting off the final clause as Mark's comment that Jesus has declared all foods clean.
Aramaic English New Testament*	Because it does not enter into his heart, rather into his belly and is cast out by excretion, which purifies all the food. *Translated from original Aramaic Peshitta texts instead of Greek.
Darby	because it does not enter into his heart but into his belly, and goes out into the draught, purging all meats?
Douay–Rheims Bible	Because it entereth not into his heart, but goeth into the belly, and goeth out into the privy, purging all meats?

Translation	Mark 7:19 Interpretation
Latin Vulgate	quia non introit in cor eius sed in ventrem et in secessum exit purgans omnes escas (or, "because not go the heart his but the belly and the draft out purging all food", word-for-word via translate. google.com)
Murdock New Testament	For it doth not enter into his heart, but into his belly, and is thrown into the digestive process, which carries off all that is eaten.
Tyndale	because it entrith not in to his hert but into ye belly: and goeth out into the draught that porgeth oute all meates.
Webster	Because it entereth not into his heart, but into the belly, and goeth out into the draught, purging all kinds of food.
World English Bible	because it doesn't go into his heart, but into his stomach, then into the latrine, thus purifying all foods[a]?" World English Bible Footnote: a. Mark 7:19 or, "making all foods clean". NU ends Jesus' direct quote and question after "latrine", ending the verse with "Thus he declared all foods clean."
Wycliffe Bible	for it hath not entered into his heart, but into the womb, and beneath it goeth out, purging all meats.
Young's Literal Translation	because it doth not enter into his heart, but into the belly, and into the drain it doth go out, purifying all the meats.

Per the examples presented in Table 4 above, which are based on inferring all words from Mark 7:19 to be from Jesus, the majority of the fourteen interpretations translate the Greek verb καθαρίζω (katharizō)[183]

---

183 Strong's G2511

as "purging," which is best representative of the context discussing the human digestive process. Moreover, the amount of creative addenda in Table 4 is kept to a minimum, with an average of four English words to replace the four words from the original Greek.

Unfortunately, the Table 4 translations above are a far cry from the majority of translations included in Table 5, which assume that Jesus finished speaking early, and that the remaining four words of the original Mark 7:19 Greek verse are attributed to Mark's commentary, where he was annotating the Gospel text.

TABLE 5—
MARK 7:19 TRANSLATED AS JESUS'
WORDS PLUS COMMENTARY

Translation	Mark 7:19 Interpretation
New International Version [#1]	For it doesn't go into his heart but into his stomach, and then out of his body." *(In saying this, Jesus declared all foods "clean.")*
American Standard Version	because it goeth not into his heart, but into his belly, and goeth out into the draught? *This he said, making all meats clean.*
Amplified Bible	Since it does not reach and enter his heart but [only his] digestive tract, and so passes on [into the place designed to receive waste]?" *Thus He was making and declaring all foods [ceremonially] clean [that is, abolishing the ceremonial distinctions of the Levitical Law].*
Basic Bible in English	Because it goes not into the heart but into the stomach, and goes out with the waste? *He said this, making all food clean.*
Christian Community Bible	Since it enters, not the heart but the stomach and is finally passed out." *Thus Jesus declared that all foods are clean.*

Translation	Mark 7:19 Interpretation
Common English Bible (#8)	That's because it doesn't enter into the heart but into the stomach, and it goes out into the sewer." *By saying this, Jesus declared that no food could contaminate a person in God's sight.*
Complete Jewish Bible	For it doesn't go into his heart but into his stomach, and it passes out into the latrine." *(Thus he declared all foods ritually clean.)*
Contemporary English Version	It doesn't go into your heart, but into your stomach, and then out of your body." *By saying this, Jesus meant that all foods were fit to eat.*
Easy-to-Read Version	Food does not go into a person's mind. It goes into the stomach. Then it goes out of the body." *(When Jesus said this, he meant there is no food that is wrong for people to eat.)*
English Standard Version (#5)	since it enters not his heart but his stomach, and is expelled?" *(Thus he declared all foods clean.)*
Expanded Bible	[Because] It does not go into the mind [heart], but into the stomach. Then it goes out of the body [into the sewer/latrine]." *(When Jesus said this, he meant that no longer was any food unclean for people to eat.)* [or, *(In this way, Jesus cleansed all food.)*]
God's Word Translation	It doesn't go into his thoughts but into his stomach and then into a toilet." *(By saying this, Jesus declared all foods acceptable.)*
Good News Translation	because it does not go into your heart but into your stomach and then goes on out of the body." *(In saying this, Jesus declared that all foods are fit to be eaten.)*

Translation	Mark 7:19 Interpretation
Holman Christian Standard Bible [(#7)]	For it doesn't go into his heart but into the stomach and is eliminated."[a] (As a result, He made all foods clean.[b]) Holman Footnotes: a. Mark 7:19 Lit goes out into the toilet. b. Mark 7:19 Other mss read "is eliminated, making all foods clean."
International Standard Version	Because it doesn't go into his heart but into his stomach, and is expelled as waste." *(By this he declared all foods clean.)*
Knox Bible	because it travels, not into his heart, but into the belly, and so finds its way into the sewer? *Thus he declared all meat to be clean,*
The Message	Jesus said, "Are you being willfully stupid? Don't you see that what you swallow can't contaminate you? It doesn't enter your heart but your stomach, works its way through the intestines, and is finally flushed." *(That took care of dietary quibbling; Jesus was saying that all foods are fit to eat.)*
Names of God	It doesn't go into his thoughts but into his stomach and then into a toilet." *(By saying this, Yeshua declared all foods acceptable.)*
New American Standard Bible (#10)	because it does not go into his heart, but into his stomach, and is eliminated?" *(Thus He declared all foods clean.)*
New Century Version	It does not go into the mind, but into the stomach. Then it goes out of the body." *(When Jesus said this, he meant that no longer was any food unclean for people to eat.)*

Translation	Mark 7:19 Interpretation
New International Reader's Version (#6)	It doesn't go into the heart. It goes into the stomach. Then it goes out of the body." *In saying this, Jesus was calling all foods "clean."*
New Living Translation (#3)	Food doesn't go into your heart, but only passes through the stomach and then goes into the sewer." *(By saying this, he declared that every kind of food is acceptable in God's eyes.)*
New Life Version	It does not go into his heart, but into his stomach and then on out of his body." *In this way, He was saying that all food is clean.*
New Revised Standard Version	since it enters, not the heart but the stomach, and goes out into the sewer?" *(Thus he declared all foods clean.)*
NRSV (Catholic)	since it enters, not the heart but the stomach, and goes out into the sewer?' *(Thus he declared all foods clean.)*
New World Translation	since it passes, not into [his] heart, but into [his] intestines, and it passes out into the sewer?" *Thus he declared all foods clean.*
Revised Standard Version	since it enters, not his heart but his stomach, and so passes on?" *(Thus he declared all foods clean.)*
Worldwide English New Testament	It does not go into his heart, but into his stomach, and then it goes out of the body." *By saying this, Jesus meant that food does not make a person dirty.*

Translations for Every Appetite

As the 42 English translations tabulated in Tables 2 and 3 above are compared with original Greek texts as included on page 18 of chapter 1, it becomes evident that all versions that interpret the last four words of the Mark 7:19 verse (e.g. "purging all the meats") as gospel author commentary (namely the latter 66.6%, as cited in Table 5) are translated with a strong dispensational slant and unclean bias. Moreover, most of these Table 5 translations also seem to interject a sizeable amount of translator commentary on what is assumed to be Mark's commentary. In fact, translations in Table 5 use an average of ten English words to replace the four words from the original Greek—compared to a humble average of four English words per the translations presented in Table 4, where all words are assumed to be a word-for-word continuation of Jesus' teaching.

Moreover, as Table 5 translations populate the conclusion of Mark 7:19 with superfluous verbs, subjects, objects, and adjectives, the texts begin to assume a host of different meanings. Rather than having the digestive tract as the subject performing a function like "cleansing" or "purging," as the lone Greek καθαρίζω (katharizō)[184] action verb should imply, many Table 5 translations transform the verb into an adjective, adding it to the end of the verse, and using it to describe the "food" subsequent to the digestion. Also, in place of the "cleansing" verb, most of the Table 5 translations insert the verb "declared" or "made" in its place, along with "Jesus" as the subject of conversation. Even though "Jesus declared" does not appear in the original Greek, these two words are nevertheless routinely added within these creative Table 5 interpretations and translations, implying that Mark was invoking Jesus' authority or power to redefine or transform all foods to be "clean," as he commented on Jesus' earlier words—supposedly clarifying what Jesus really intended to convey.

Further implying that Jesus was involved in a food conversion process of some sort, most translations go so far as to describe all "food" as "clean," "pure," "acceptable," "fitting," morally neutral, or even edible—forgetting that earlier in the verse, Jesus was concluding his description of a bodily waste handling process, alluding to the latrine or the process of expelling unclean human defecation. Some translations insert weaker verbs, such as "meant," "said," or "called," to imply a

---

184 Strong's G2511

more reason-oriented interpretation, suggesting that Jesus was merely using his special insight, superior intellect, or power of observation to reclassify foods contrary to Moses.

Still other translations are far more ambitious and original, boldly inserting the verb "abolishing" in conjunction with "ceremony," "ritual," or "Levitical law"—even though the original Greek makes no such references whatsoever! In accordance with the Table 5 texts illustrated in tables above, it is clear that the translations read more like doctrinal statements, proving that there are indeed translations to appease all appetites, be they theological or culinary. Some translations appear to be nothing less than novel attempts to avoid copyright infringement or attain a unique status for the sake of copyright claim, in which the final meaning of the translation is of secondary importance.

Translations Reconsidered and Pursued

While this book is hardly meant to serve as an endorsement for antiquated English translations, as an English Bible buyer's guide, or as a comprehensive critique of Bible translations, it is nevertheless intended to stimulate readers into reconsidering the validity of translations that would otherwise be accepted at face value, or as divinely inspired. Hopefully, at a minimum, this book will inspire readers to question the numerous assumptions and interpretations on which their English translations are based—assumptions which in turn have formulated their traditions and doctrines. For example, what if English Bible translations pertaining to eternal salvation doctrines are as adulterated as simple dining doctrines? Clearly, the translations and interpretations of others are instrumental in shaping knowledge, beliefs, and faith— perhaps far more than most people ever thought possible!

Fortunately, many Bible truths are able to rise above even the worst of translations, even though translation problems may be numerous and blatant. For this very reason, Christians from around the world have expended a great deal of time and effort in order to obtain the best Bible translation available in their native tongue, benefiting greatly from Bible translations. Moreover, over the centuries some have even risked life and limb to translate, to acquire, or to even read the Bible in English.

Today however, after literally hundreds of different English translations have been penned or typeset by an equally vast number of individuals and religious organizations, many people are presented with a very different problem—they want to know which English version to read! They want an accurate translation, one which they can trust as divinely inspired. They want an unbiased translation, free of religious dogma and untainted by political agendas, one that conveys divine authority and instructions without partiality. They want a package that captures the essence of the ancient culture and the spirit of the original text. They want to know what the Bible actually says—not what somebody else thinks it means. And finally, they want it at the snap of a finger, or in today's terms, at the click of a mouse.

Translation Complications

Of course, even where scholars' intentions are completely noble, Bible translation is a challenging endeavor often wrought with controversy. At best, translation is an imperfect art complicated by the asymmetrical mechanics of two unique languages; it is anything but an absolute and objective science. In converting a message from one language into another, there is simply no assurance that all ideas, social norms, idiomatic expressions, slang, or even words can be directly transmitted in a like-for-like manner or on a word-for-word basis. So not surprisingly, it is inevitable that translations will take on different words and even different meanings as people of differing perspectives wrestle with various linguistic idiosyncrasies and cultural barriers.

Obviously, individual perspective is guaranteed to further influence and complicate translations. As proposed by the famous Indian parable, a blind man below the head of an elephant might describe a snake like trunk, whereas a blind man surveying a leg might compare the elephant to a tree. Although neither man is incorrect in his perspective, neither man is completely correct either, as neither man can perceive or describe the entire animal. As aptly and eloquently concluded by American poet John Godfrey Saxe,

So oft in theologic wars,
The disputants, I ween,
Rail on in utter ignorance
Of what each other mean,
And prate about an Elephant
Not one of them has seen![185]

Bible translation could be likened to "The Blindmen and the Elephant" poem, as two different individuals might interpret and translate a single verse differently without being incorrect, each expressing a part of a greater truth beyond their own limited perception. Furthermore, personal experiences, passions, aptitudes, and knowledge bases will contribute to differing individual perspectives, thereby influencing how one translator will interpret or prioritize key words or phrases relative to another translator. Where translations are made by more than one individual, multiple interpretations might be blended together in order to create a more complete description. However, such compromises can also produce odd and incompatible heterogeneous amalgamations. Doing justice to neither viewpoint, thinking that their eyes have been opened, what they envision together might easily be mistaken for a snake perched in a tree!

Translation Arguments

Because believers intuitively understand that Bible translation quality is of paramount importance, they zealously guard their preferred English rendition as God's Word with great passion and even prejudice—often committing to a single translation. In some cases, people may acquire a strong allegiance to a given version simply as a result of personal familiarity and time in study. Others will

---

185 http://www.noogenesis.com/pineapple/blind_men_elephant.html

confine themselves to a particular translation because of third party endorsement, as directed by a parent, pastor, respected teacher, or religious institution. Some prefer to hold fast to their Bible translation as a matter of tradition, reserving a special place in their hearts for texts that sound more established, timeless, or poetic. Still others prefer a contemporary English translation, assuming that translation into the vernacular will maximize their comprehension as a reader; some also assume that new translations represent the summation or accumulation of knowledge, and that the end result is therefore of the best possible scholarship. Finally, there are those who dogmatically believe that their translation was divinely inspired, protected from any possible error in human interpretation, perhaps because the thought of God depriving them of a perfect translation within their own tongue is an idea too abhorrent to accept.

Unfortunately, where strong loyalties are present, great arguments are sure to follow, contributing in turn to battles and factions, many of which divide congregations. These congregations are often comprised of members individually oblivious to the variants in English translation, and equally unaware of what the original language conveys. It is as disconcerting as it is ironic that such caustic fruit should be the end result of hundreds of English Bible translation attempts.

Given this trend toward argument and division, perhaps it is time to reconsider asking "which Bible version is best?", reverting back to a different question of greater importance, "should the Bible have ever been translated at all?"

Translations Degradation

While questioning the prudence of Bible translation might initially sound absurd and even hostile to Jesus' "go ye therefore" Great Commission, it is of some significance that the Bible itself never once instructed its audience to make written translations of its content into other languages.[186] In fact, both Old and New Testament texts seem to discourage the practice of creating written translations altogether, given that the translation process inherently introduces all sorts of additions, subtractions, and amendments to the original texts, just as the English quotes at the opening of this chapter discourage.[187]

Translation of Bible texts into any language ultimately requires compromise; amendments, shortages, and surpluses of all sorts— regardless of method or destination language—are required for translation. Even in cases where a direct word-for-word translation is attempted, such translation runs the risk of not conveying complete ideas because languages differ in syntaxes, logical construction, and vocabularies. In comparison, thought-for-thought or paraphrase translations are hardly without liabilities of their own, for they require the changing of words and omission of essential details. Furthermore, every language has its own set of rules and quirks; things like idioms, metaphors, synonyms, homonyms, rhyme, cultural allusions, preposition usage, and wordplay are not readily captured in translation, yet each contribute uniquely to the meaning of a verse. Because the ancient Scriptures are replete with such intricacies, it is logical to conclude that any translation of the original will result in some level of degradation of meaning or a loss of information, regardless of translation method or diligence on the part of the translator. In fact, it would be absurd to propose anything to the contrary. A perfect translation is like a square circle, or like a kosher lobster dinner; it is a logical fallacy.

Translation Objections

While proposing to apply the aforementioned "don't add to" and "don't subtract from" commandments to the tradition of Bible translation may sound radical and unwarranted—even heretical among evangelical circles and Bible societies—there are actually precedents

---

186 1 Corinthians 14 endorsed oral translation, not lasting permanent translations to original texts.
187 Deuteronomy 4:2, Proverbs 30:6, Jeremiah 8:8, Revelation 22:18–19

established in biblical texts that seem to oppose written translation of the Scriptures. For example, referring to the original Hebrew Scriptures, Jesus himself insisted that all of the "jots and tittles" would remain relevant and in effect until "heaven and earth disappeared."[188] In this statement, Jesus was referring to the smallest letters, decorative markings, and textual anomalies of the Hebrew text, which are uniquely added to select sections of the Scriptures, conveying hints and deeper meanings.[189] Obviously, translators have failed to capture such jots or tittles throughout all of the hundreds of English Bible versions created to date, even though Jesus spoke plainly of the Hebrew precision and deeper meanings embedded within the original texts.

Jesus was not unique in this 'revert to the original language' thinking. The Jerusalem council of Acts was rightfully compelled to refer the new Gentile believers to the synagogues on the Sabbath, where they could hear Scripture read in the original language.[190] Likewise, as a great prophet and priest, Ezra grieved as the exiles returned from pagan Babylon, specifically because they were speaking foreign languages and had become estranged from their native Hebrew tongue. Surely, this account suggests that Ezra did not want to translate the Bible into the language of Ashdod or other foreign tongues; instead, Ezra wanted the exiles returning to Israel to return also to the original language of the Bible.[191] As priest and prophet, Ezra wanted the people to see things clearly, and to see for themselves. He did not want the restored nation to be forced into reliance on dozens of different translations catered to each man's dialect, only to hear them bickering over translation supremacy; neither did Ezra want to spend the remainder of his days listening to two blind men attempt to describe an elephant.

Should believers conform their thinking and culture to the Scriptures, or should the Scriptures be conformed to the people to accommodate their thinking and cultures? Clearly, both imperative statements and narratives in both Hebrew and Greek canons underscore

---

188 Matthew 5:18
189 http://scrolls4all.com/Scribal_Oddities.php
190 Acts 15:21
191 Nehemiah 13:24

the problems inherent in translation. Rather than having the original language converted imperfectly to satisfy the reader's ignorance, dialect, experiences, and appetites, the preferred approach—even in Bible translations demonstrating strong dispensational biases—is for people to convert themselves to understand the original divinely inspired language, lest they mistake their inferior and imperfect translations for the complete and perfect truth.

Translation Dependency

Since the time of Shakespeare, the English idiom "it's all Greek to me" has been used to describe nearly anything which is not readily understandable. While on one hand the expression is useful for confessing personal ignorance, on the other hand, depending on context and vocal inflection, the expression might also express helplessness, condone apathy, or profess a crippling attitude. Not only might it say, "I don't know," but it also might coincidentally suggest, "I couldn't ever possibly know," or possibly "I don't care." Given this versatility, the "it's all Greek to me" expression becomes a convenient way to respond when confronted with ancient Bible languages.

While many religious organizations have been diligent throughout the generations in dispatching handfuls of scholars to study the ancient languages in institutions of higher learning, it is fair to say that these same organizations have been equally negligent in raising their congregants to comparable levels of proficiency. Rather than teaching the congregants how to translate and understand the texts, they rely almost exclusively on translations, interpreting and translating for the congregant on rare occasions. In so doing, they intimidate and even stifle their audience, imposing a "can't do" attitude on them. Instead of encouraging members to explore the texts in their original languages, many religious institutions instead promote systems of dependency, whereby congregants are encouraged to attend as passive bystanders and without accountability, in this way subconsciously encouraging the masses to remain in a perpetual state of infancy. Unfortunately, the end result of such passive approaches and stifling environments is the subsistence feeding of congregants, who, as Paul put it, are "not ready for solid meat."[192] Such institutions lead congregants to believe that there exists only one cow on the entire earth from which to derive milk, thus creating a perception of artificial scarcity—only to justify astronomical milk prices in excess of market value. Accepting a mere ration of milk, believers are not introduced to the herds of cows, sheep, and goats aboard Noah's Ark—all of which are capable of producing both milk and meat. Instead, they are taught to "kill and eat" *anything*.

Translation Alternatives

Today, there are numerous alternatives to Bible translations and interpretations; but they are seldom, if ever, made available or promoted by status quo religious institutions via weekly service schedules or academic curriculums. Most church services and programs do not offer biblical language study programs, and the same can be said of grade school and high school curriculums—even among private schools run by religious institutions. Congregants are given church catechisms in the place of concordances, directed to constitutions instead of language lexicons, and memorize English doctrines and creeds over ancient texts.

By the time the average American Christian student completes high school, that student might have attended in excess of 20,000 hours of school curriculum, along with 750 hours of church services. To put this in perspective, it would take that student just three new words per day over the course of their curriculum to learn every word in the entire Hebrew Bible.

Young students are taught that things like art, science, geometry, math, penmanship, social studies, history, music, home economics, English, and religious doctrine are important. Yet by means of omission, students are inherently also taught that understanding God's word in original biblical languages is far less important than all other fields of

---

192 1 Corinthians 3:2, Hebrews 5:12, 13, Genesis 7, Leviticus 11

study, and this during the time they are at their prime potential for language absorption and acclimation.

Though biblical language study tools are available for free in this information age, it remains inevitable that individuals, families, and institutions will remain unable to reason beyond translations until they make it a priority to employ such resources. Until knowledge is pursued, it cannot be attained. Thus, as long as religious institutions continue to remain indifferent towards ancient language education, the only true alternatives to imperfect translations will be individual time and commitment. However, such investment in knowledge promises to return something priceless—both in this world and the next.

Translating Ignorance into Consequences

While agnostics might hope that ignorance of the truth will somehow cover a multitude of sins, Scripture testifies to the contrary. In fact, ignorance is said to be a precursor to destruction. Speaking on God's behalf, the prophet Hosea said of Israel,

My people are destroyed for lack of knowledge... (Hos 4:6a).

Hosea wasn't speaking simply about a lack of a conventional education—or about ignorance of a particular church doctrine. Instead, he was speaking specifically about God's law, and the deliberate rejection of knowledge. Hosea continued,

...because you have rejected knowledge, I also reject you as my priests; because you have ignored the law of your God, I also will ignore your children" (Hos 4:6b).

Although Hosea did not itemize a litany of dietary law transgressions as he rebuked the Israelites over two thousand years ago, it would seem that the principles of his prophecies remain directly transferrable to this generation. After all, youth today are students of algebra, chemistry, calculus, and even biology—yet they don't know even know how many cows were aboard Noah's ark. They are not told the first thing about defining food according to the Bible, specifically as it has been outlined in Moses' law. They fail to understand how failure to observe these laws might have consequences, even resulting in their own demise. People *are destroyed* by eating unclean and defiled food in complete ignorance!

Translating Science into Knowledge

Centuries ago, before science became synonymous with natural philosophy, and before the scientific method became the predominant approach to the study of the natural world, the term science was used in a larger and more comprehensive sense. The word science was derived from a Latin term, which more generically means knowledge. Thus Hosea's famous prophetic claim might just as legitimately read,

"My people are destroyed for lack of science."

Science isn't the only term that has assumed a different meaning since the King James Bible was first distributed. The animal types that the Bible refers to as "unclean," science might refer to today as "biohazards." It is for this reason that the "unclean" animal varieties, consisting of scavengers, carnivores, and omnivores, are not qualified as "food" for people according to Bible texts. For good reason, God forbade the Israelites to eat unclean things such as clams, crabs, mussels, oysters, scallops, lobsters, shrimp, squid, octopus, eels, sharks, catfish, camels, rodents, rabbits, horses, pigs, boars, bears, dogs, cats, frogs, reptiles, worms, beetles, flies, or scavenging birds of prey.

Although the extent of Moses' knowledge in the field of biology is unknown, God knew by design that these same "unclean" animals host or accumulate a variety of harmful parasites, bacteria, biotoxins, carcinogens, and viruses, based largely on their diets. The list of biohazards transmitted by unclean animals includes parasitic worms like anisakiasis, gnathostomiasis, hookworms, nybelinia surmenicola, pinworms, roundworms, taenia solium (i.e., pork tapeworm), and trichinosis or trichinellosis;[193] bacteria such as cholera, E. coli, listeria monocytogenes, salmonella, staphylococcus aureus, vibrio cholerae, vibrio parahaemolyticus, yersinia enterocolitica;[194] biotoxins such as Amnesic shellfish poisoning (ASP), Neurotoxic shellfish poisoning (NSP), and Paralytic shellfish poisoning (PSP);[195] carcinogens like DDT, PCB's, and heavy metals;[196] or viruses like Hepatitis A, Hepatitis E, or the Norwalk virus.[197] Knowing what might reside in the blood of unclean animals, God not only told people to abstain from eating these things—he even directed them to avoid touching the carcasses of such animals, understanding it to be a health hazard, both private and communicable, and thus a "sin."[198]

Long before the Center for Disease Control (CDC) was formed and various research on unclean foods was published, God understood the

---

193 http://www.cdc.gov/parasites/anisakiasis/faqs.html,
http://www.cdc.gov/parasites/gnathostoma/faqs.html,
http://www.cfsph.iastate.edu/Factsheets/pdfs/hookworms.pdf,
http://dailyparasite.blogspot.com/2010/08/august-8-nybelinia-surmenicola.html,
http://en.wikipedia.org/wiki/Pork,
http://www.cdc.gov/parasites/taeniasis/gen_info/faqs.html,
http://www.cdc.gov/parasites/trichinellosis/gen_info/faqs.html,
http://www.cdc.gov/parasites/resources/pdf/npi_cysticercosis.pdf
194 http://www.cdc.gov/cholera/general/, http://en.wikipedia.org/wiki/Pork,
http://www.ncbi.nlm.nih.gov/pubmed/16834586,
http://www.ncbi.nlm.nih.gov/pubmed/2243182,
http://www.cdc.gov/nczved/divisions/dfbmd/diseases/vibriop/#what http://www.
cdc.gov/ncidod/dbmd/diseaseinfo/yersinia_g.htm
195 http://www.cdc.gov/ncidod/dbmd/diseaseinfo/marinetoxins_g.htm#whatare,
http://www.cdc.gov/niosh/ershdb/EmergencyResponseCard_29750019.html
196 http://www.atsdr.cdc.gov/phs/phs.asp?id=79&tid=20, http://www.atsdr.cdc.gov/
phs/phs.asp?id=139&tid=26, http://www.atsdr.cdc.gov/phs/phs.asp?id=46&tid=15,
http://www.atsdr.cdc.gov/hac/pha/pha.asp?docid=1341&pg=1
197 http://en.wikipedia.org/wiki/Hepatitis_A, http://www.cdc.gov/norovirus/
198 Leviticus 11:8

diseases and various consequences associated with eating unclean things. He knew that eating substances and microorganisms contained within unclean animals could result in short term problems like abdominal pain, nausea, vomiting, diarrhea, fever, temperature reversal, headaches, excess tiredness, lack of appetite, dizziness, disorientation, floating sensations, numbness, or tingling in the mouth, arms, and legs. He understood that eating unclean foods might even result in symptoms such as loss of coordination, permanent short-term memory loss, focal weakness or paralysis, vision loss, blindness, muscle paralysis, seizures, adult onset epilepsy, respiratory failure, severe nerve pain, paralysis, decreased consciousness, comas, and even death.

Dispensational Translation Rejection

In rejecting God's dietary commandments as given through Moses, dispensational theologians not only reject the goodness of God as a law giver, but they propagate unholy and unkosher Bible doctrines through misinterpretations and mistranslations, demonstrating a gross lack of knowledge. They promote a backward theology where white is black and black is white, and where right is wrong and wrong is right. They propose that Jesus avoided unclean animals—as described by Moses—strictly for purposes of religious ceremony, short term messianic obligation, or for the sake of manmade traditions. They insist that the dietary law is "done away with," encouraging others to share in the sin of Adam and Eve. They eat foods forbidden by Moses, not acknowledging that sin is defined by the law and that "the wages of sin is death."[199]

Equipped with the knowledge of Scripture in its full contexts and original languages, no honest or reasonable scientifically-minded 21st century individual with a simple understanding of biological life would conclude that Jesus came to earth two thousand years ago to expel all parasites and biohazards from the entire planet. Jesus didn't convert non-food animals into food—either by messianic miracle or by authoritative proclamation. There is no biblical or other historical record

199 Romans 6:23, Romans 7:7

describing how the various biohazards of Jesus' time either transformed or vanished before, during, or after his crucifixion. Jesus did not, and would not, dine on dispensational doctrines or translations; he would reject them as unclean.

Translating Commandments into Love

On the contrary, Jesus' diet, as defined by God through Moses, makes perfect sense from both a biblical and a scientific standpoint. By pairing simple science with a moral reverence for life, it becomes obvious why Moses discouraged even physical contact with biohazard-carrying animal carcasses, why Daniel would not share his kitchen with abominable creatures, and why Peter would not put any defiled food on his tablecloth or bring any unclean food to his lips. Likewise, Paul would not eat unclean creatures if they were served to him at an unbeliever's house; and if they were placed before him, he would indeed raise questions of conscience. He would respond like Peter and Ezekiel; he would consider them to be unclean in and of themselves, irrespective of pagan temple or idol proximity. God reminded Noah to eat clean foods as he disembarked from the Ark, just as he blessed Adam and Eve with the same dominion and diet back in the Garden of Eden.

It is more than the least of all human commandments to *EAT LIKE JESUS*; it is among the first of all human commandments. It is an act of obedience. It is a path to self-preservation, and it is a way to keep one's neighbor from harm. It is an act of love to treat the body like a temple of the Holy Spirit and to guard it from debilitating disease.

Beyond Dietary Translations

With respect to religious reform, *EAT LIKE JESUS* might be likened to the tip of an iceberg. Apart from a few simple food-related doctrines, what other great truths lurk beneath the surface of other religious traditions and dispensational dogmas? What if Christians wholeheartedly revered God's other commandments given through Moses, as Jesus did? What if believers began to see Moses' law as a gift of love from God, rather than as an expression of God's curse? What would the rest of the Bible look like if translated into English with a kosher view instead of a dispensational one? What other knowledge do the original Bible texts contain beneath the translators' many assumptions and interpretations?

What would it look like, if the Christian church set aside dispensational dogma, religious traditions, and secondhand translations, returning to Kosher Christianity in every aspect of life? How might it affect other fields of study and occupations, such as agriculture, medicine, hygiene, government, law enforcement, economics, commerce, real estate, education, or family life? What about Christian doctrines—such as salvation, grace, repentance, forgiveness, redemption, atonement, sacrifice, communion, or baptism? What would these things look like apart from the dogma, traditions, and mistranslations? How do they shape religious thought and what effects might they have on individual behavior or society as a whole?

These questions are left for the reader's consideration and investigation—or perhaps another book.

> "Come now, let us reason together," says the LORD. "Though your sins are like scarlet, they shall be as white as snow; though they are red as crimson, they shall be like wool." (Isa. 1:18)

Chapter 5 Notes